RENAL DIET
COOKBOOK FOR BEGINNERS

Endless Culinary Explorations: Easy and Nutrient-Conscious Dishes Tailored to You.

Discover a World of Tasty, Low- Sodium, Low-Potassium, Low- Phosphorus Recipes for Healthy Kidneys

SERENA HARPER

3 SPECIAL BONUSES
BONUS 1: Renal-Friendly Festive Menu
BONUS 2: Renal-Friendly Dining Out Guide
BONUS 3: Renal-Friendly Guide of Supplements and Herbs

If you find *Renal Diet Cookbook for Beginners* helpful and inspiring, we'd be immensely grateful for your kind words in an Amazon review.

<u>Your feedback means the world to us</u> and plays a crucial role in supporting our small publishing house. Thank you for being a valued part of our community and for sharing the love of good health and great food!

Simply **scan the QR code provided** and effortlessly contribute to our community of readers.

The Table of
CONTENTS

Introduction: Understanding CKD and its Emotional Impact

You have two small organs called kidneys in your back, just below your ribs. They're about the same size as your fist. Inside each kidney, there are tiny parts called nephrons. These nephrons help clean your blood. There are lots of them, about a million!

Your kidneys do important jobs like getting rid of waste, bad stuff, and extra water from your body. They also make sure there are the right salts and minerals in your blood. They even release special chemicals to control your blood pressure, help your blood carry oxygen, and keep your bones strong. All the waste and extra water your kidneys take out turn into something called urine. This urine travels through tubes called ureters and ends up in a bag-like thing called your bladder. Your bladder holds onto the urine till you go to the bathroom.

What is Chronic Kidney Disease?

Chronic kidney disease (CKD) is when your kidneys get hurt and can't do their job properly. Imagine your kidneys as filters in your body. They clean out bad stuff like waste and extra water from your blood. They also help your bones and blood stay healthy. But when your kidneys start to have problems, they can't clean out the waste, and it piles up in your blood.

We call it "chronic" because it happens slowly over time. CKD can even lead to kidney failure, which is really bad. Not everyone with CKD gets kidney failure, but if we don't treat it, things can get worse. Sadly, there's no magic fix for CKD, but we can do things to slow it down. When CKD gets really bad, we might need treatments like dialysis or a kidney transplant.

Here are some signs that something might be wrong with your kidneys: **pee troubles, swelling, feeling tired, itchy skin, weird tastes and breath, hard to breathe and feeling cold.**

If you notice any of these signs, it's a good idea to see a doctor. They can help you figure out if your kidneys need some extra care.

CKD unfolds in stages, discerned by the gradual decline of kidney function, measured through the glomerular filtration rate (GFR). The journey through these stages paints a narrative of diminishing kidney capacity:

Stage 1: Minimal Damage with Normal or High GFR
- GFR: >90 mL/min
- Kidney damage with standard kidney function, potentially detected by other markers.

Stage 2: Mild Loss of Kidney Function
- GFR: 60-89 mL/min
- Slightly diminished kidney function, necessitating vigilant observation to prevent progression.

Stage 3: Moderate Loss of Kidney Function
- GFR: 30-59 mL/min
- A tangible decrease in function, with physical symptoms potentially making a debut, signaling the imperative for strategic management.

Stage 4: Severe Loss of Kidney Function
- GFR: 15-29 mL/min
- Advanced kidney damage, where deliberate management strategies are pivotal to delay the advent of end-stage renal disease (ESRD).

Stage 5 or ESRD: Kidney Failure
- GFR: <15 mL/min or on dialysis
- Necessitates renal replacement therapy – dialysis or a kidney transplant – to sustain life and manage health.

Pass through these stages, it's vital to adeptly manage CKD by incorporating dietary adjustments, medication management, and lifestyle modifications, ensuring a holistic approach to mitigating complications and enhancing quality of life.

Essential Fact that Every Renal Patient Should Know

CKD is a global health concern, with its prevalence increasing over the years. According to the World Health Organization (WHO), CKD affects around 10% of the world's population. It is 9th leading causes of death in US, affecting more than 37 million people. It is more prevalent in older adults, but it can occur at any age. Early detection and management are critical to slowing its progression.

One out of every three grown-ups in America has a big chance of getting kidney problems, but most of them can't tell when something is wrong with their kidneys. One out of every nine grown-ups in America actually has kidney problems, but they don't even know it!

At first, kidney problems don't make you feel bad. You won't notice anything till your kidneys are really hurt. Usually, people don't have any signs till it's too late. The only way to find out if your kidneys are okay is to do special blood and pee tests.

Main Causes

There are many reasons why someone might develop Chronic Kidney Disease (CKD). The primary causes are Diabetes and Hypertension, accounting for approximately 75% of CKD causes.

Other reasons why CKD might develop are: Glomerulonephritis, Interstitial Nephritis, Recurrent Kidney Infections or Inherited Kidney Diseases. It's important to take care of your overall health and manage conditions mainly like diabetes and high blood pressure to reduce the risk of CKD.

Other Diseases and Related Complications

Chronic Kidney Disease (CKD) adversely impacts various health aspects, leading to several related complications and associated health issues. Notably, it amplifies the risk of cardiovascular problems, like heart disease and stroke, due to its role in blood pressure regulation and maintaining electrolyte and fluid balance. CKD can also induce anemia by hampering the kidneys' ability to produce erythropoietin, a hormone crucial for red blood cell production, leading to fatigue and weakness. Furthermore, it poses a significant threat to bone health by disrupting the body's calcium and phosphorus balance, potentially resulting in weakened bones and increasing fracture risk. Additionally, CKD might cause fluid retention, manifesting as swelling in various body parts, due to the kidneys' diminished ability to expel extra sodium and water, possibly elevating blood pressure and damaging other organs in severe instances.

The foods tailored for CKD do more than just aid your kidneys—they profoundly reshape your gut microbiome. With recent studies emphasizing the powerful symbiotic relationship between a balanced gut and optimal kidney function, there's never been a more crucial time to prioritize dietary choices. Dive into the intriguing gut-kidney connection and let your diet do wonders!

Facing the Emotional Challenges: From Fears of Dialysis to Dietary Changes

Dealing with kidney problems can be emotionally challenging. The thought of needing dialysis can be scary. It's important to address these fears and make necessary dietary changes.

Firstly, please know you are not alone in this and understand that it's natural to feel anxious about dialysis. Sharing your apprehensions with loved ones or even joining a support group can make a world of difference. Listening to others who have walked this path can bring solace and understanding.

When ready, take a deep breath and immerse yourself in understanding dialysis. The more you know about it, the more you'll see its potential benefits and how it strives to give you a life worth cherishing.

Diet, while seemingly a small piece of the puzzle, plays a crucial role in this journey. Seek out a renal dietitian; their expertise can help craft a diet that not only suits your health needs but also indulges your palate. Dietary shifts can be a gateway to not only preserving kidney function but also discovering new delicious meals.

According to a study in the Journal of Renal Nutrition, CKD patients who adhere to a kidney-friendly diet can experience a significant improvement in the efficiency of their dialysis treatments! Your plate doesn't just carry food; it holds the power to optimize your dialysis sessions. Each bite can be a step closer to better health. Harness the potential of your meals and elevate your dialysis experience!

Stay mindful of your hydration levels, and be cautious with certain minerals like salt, potassium, and phosphorus. While this might mean bidding adieu to some of your favorites, there's a world of scrumptious alternatives awaiting you.

Life's beauty lies in balance. Pair your treatment with gentle exercises and embrace practices that soothe your soul. Together, they'll pave the way for a more harmonious, hopeful tomorrow.

1. The Basics of the Renal Diet

Benefits of Renal Diet

- **Control Blood Pressure:** It helps regulate blood pressure, reducing the risk of heart problems.
- **Manage Fluid Levels:** It helps control body fluids, avoiding swelling and shortness of breath.
- **Limit Waste Buildup:** It reduces waste buildup in the blood, which can make you feel sick.
- **Preserve Kidney Function:** It can slow down the damage to your kidneys, helping them work better for longer.
- **Minimize Protein:** It limits protein intake to ease the burden on your kidneys.
- **Balance Electrolytes:** It helps maintain healthy levels of minerals like sodium, potassium, and phosphorus.
- **Boost Energy:** It can improve energy levels and overall well-being.
- **Reduce Toxin Buildup:** It lessens the accumulation of toxins in the body, preventing complications.
- **Control Blood Sugar:** It aids in managing blood sugar levels, especially if you have diabetes alongside CKD.
- **Maintain a Healthy Weight:** It helps with weight management, which is crucial for kidney health.
- Remember, a renal diet should be personalized, so it's essential to work with a healthcare professional or a registered dietitian to create a plan that suits your specific needs.

Recent studies reveal a compelling link between diet and well-being. CKD patients who follow a nutrient conscious diet not only have a 30% slower progression rate but also report a 25% increase in overall mood and energy levels. The power of diet transcends physical health—it's a mood-lifter, too! Dive into the science of eating right for holistic wellness

Micronutrients: Potassium, Phosphorus and Sodium

The treatment and dietary recommendations for CKD can vary depending on the stage of the disease. Please note that specific dietary and medical guidance should be provided by a healthcare professional, as individual circumstances and requirements can differ. However, here is a general daily guidance table for specific stages of CKD:

Element	Stage 1	Stage 2	Stage 3	Stage 4
Sodium	<2.3g	<2.3g	<2.0g	<1.5g
Calcium	1.0-1.3g	1.0-1.3g	0.8-1.2g	0.8-1.0g
Phosphorus	<0.8g	<0.8g	<0.8g	<0.6g
Potassium	2.0-3.0g	2.0-3.0g	2.0-3.0g	2.0-2.5g
Proteins	0.8 g/kg*	0.8 g/kg*	0.8 g/kg*	0.6 g/kg*

*referring to grams of protein per kilogram of body weight.

Sodium

Sodium is a kind of mineral found in many natural foods. Some people might mix up sodium with salt, but they're a bit different. Salt is actually made up of sodium and another substance called chloride. The things we eat can have salt in them, or they can have sodium in other forms. Foods that are made in factories often have more sodium because they include salt to them.

People with kidney problems need to be careful about how much sodium they eat. If they have too much sodium, their kidneys can't get rid of it well. This extra sodium and liquid can build up in their body and make blood pressure go up.

How can people with kidney problems keep an eye on how much sodium they eat?
- Check in the labels how much sodium is in the food.
- Pay attention to how big the serving is.
- Try to eat fresh meat instead of meat that comes in packages.
- Choose fresh fruits and vegetables, or tinned and frozen ones without added salt.
- Compare different brands and pick the ones with less sodium.
- Use spices that don't have "salt" in their name. For example, use garlic powder instead of garlic salt.
- When cooking at home, don't include salt.
- Keep the total sodium in a meal to around 400 mg, and for snacks, aim for around 150 mg.

Foods Lower in Sodium	Foods Higher in Sodium
<ul><li>Fresh Fruits</li><li>Fresh Vegetables</li><li>Homemade Soups</li><li>Unsalted Nuts and Seeds</li><li>Fresh Meat, Poultry, Fish</li><li>Fresh Herbs & Spices</li><li>Plain Rice & Pasta</li><li>Fresh Eggs</li><li>Oatmeal without Salt</li></ul>	<ul><li>Canned Vegetables</li><li>Deli Meats</li><li>Canned Soups</li><li>Fast Food Items</li><li>Frozen Meals</li><li>Soy Sauce</li><li>Bouillon Cubes</li><li>Packaged Instant Noodles</li><li>Pickled Vegetables</li><li>Pretzels and Salted Snacks</li><li>Salad dressing, marinades</li><li>Cottage cheese</li></ul>

Potassium

Potassium is a mineral that helps our heart beat regularly and our muscles work right. It's also important for keeping the right amount of fluids and electrolytes in our blood.

When our kidneys stop working well, they can't take out extra potassium, so it builds up inside us. Having too much potassium in our blood, called hyperkalemia, can cause muscles getting weak or irregular heart beating, which can even lead to hearth attack.

Here are some tips to keep your potassium levels safe:
- Only have a small amount of milk and dairy stuff, like 8 oz. a day.
- Choose fresh fruits and veggies.
- Don't use salt replacements or seasonings with potassium in them. Salt substitutes often contain potassium.
- Look at the labels on packaged foods, like tinned soups and tomato products, and stay away from things with potassium chloride.
- Pay attention to how much you eat at a time.
- Keep a journal of what you eat.
- Eat smaller portions foods high in protein at meal, like meat, poultry, beans, diary.

Foods Lower in Potassium (200 mg or less)	Foods Higher in Potassium (more than 200 mg)
• Berries(strawberries, blueberries) • Apples • Grapes • Pineapple • Cabbage • bell peppers • Green beans • Cucumber • Cauliflower • Corn • Mashrooms (fresh) • White rice • White pasta and bread • Yellow squash (without seeds)	• Oranges and Orange Juice • Bananas • Tomatoes and Tomato Products • Aprocots • Cantaloupe • Potatoes and Sweet Potatoes • Spinach and broccoli (cooked) • Beans (like kidney and navy beans) • Lentils • Dairy Products (like milk and yogurt) • Dried Fruits (like raisins and prunes) • Mashrooms (cooked) • Avocados

Potassium level is based on one serving. One serving of vegetables is ½ teacup fresh or cooked, 1 teacup raw leafy vegetables, or ½ teacup juice. One serving of fruit is one small piece; ½ teacup fresh, tinned, or cooked fruit; ¼ teacup dried fruit; or ½ teacup juice.

Phosphorus

Phosphorus is a mineral that helps our bones, tissues, and muscles. When we eat food with phosphorus, our body absorbs it and stores it in our bones.

When kidneys don't work well, the phosphorus can build up in your body and make our bones weak and cause calcium to build up in our blood vessels, lungs, eyes, and heart, which can be harmful.

How can patients watch their phosphorus intake? Phosphorus is in many foods, so his level needs to be managed:

- Eat smaller amounts of high-protein foods during meals and snacks.
- Choose fresh fruits and vegetables (keeping always an eye on your Potassium).
- Ask your doctor about using medicines called phosphate binders during meals.
- Avoid packaged foods that have extra phosphorus. Check the ingredient labels for "phosphorus" or words with "PHOS" in them (for example PyroPHOSphate)
- Keep a food diary to track what you eat.

Foods Lower in Phosphorus	Foods Higher in Phosphorus
• Rice milk (not enriched) • Apples • Fresh fruits and vegetables • Corn and rice cereals • White bread and rice • Fish	• Milk and other dairy products • Cheese • Whole grain breads • Brown rice • Oats • Bran cereals • Beans and lentils • Nuts and seeds • Fish and meat

Nutritional Needs and CKD: Proteins, Fats, Carbohydrates

Protein

Proteins are like building blocks for our body. They help us grow, fix our body parts, and keep our muscles strong. They also help make the enzymes, which help our body work, and they keep us healthy.

When our kidneys don't work well, they have trouble getting rid of waste from protein. This waste is called urea and creatinine. If we eat too much protein, these waste things can build up in our blood and make our kidneys work even worse. So, it's important to be careful with how much protein we eat if our kidneys are not working well.

A doctor or a nutrition expert can figure out how much protein is right for someone with kidney problems. They consider things like how bad the kidney problem is, how old the person is, if they're a man or a woman, and other stuff. It's important to eat just the right amount of protein that our body needs without making our kidneys work too hard. It's best to choose healthy protein foods like lean meat, chicken, fish, eggs, and dairy products.

If you are vegetarian, talk to your dietitian about how tone sure to get from plants all proteins your body needs, without impacting safe level of phosphorus and potassium.

Fats

Eating fats from food gives your body energy, helps carry certain vitamins, and helps with body jobs.

People with kidney problems have a higher chance of heart problems. Eating less bad fats can lower this chance. Bad fats, like the ones in fried and packaged foods, can make heart problems worse. People with kidney problems should eat good fats like those in avocados, olive oil, nuts, seeds, and fish. It's also important to eat the right amount of food and calories.

Do you know that extra virgin olive oil is full of anti-inflammatory compounds. Drizzling it over salads or using it in cooking can be beneficial for your kidneys.

Carbohydrates

Carbohydrates give your body energy. They help your brain, muscles, and cells work properly.

People with CKD need carbohydrates for energy, but they have to be careful. They must watch how many carbs they eat to keep their blood sugar in check, especially if they also have diabetes, which is common in CKD.

Do you know that quinoa and bulgur are not only delicious but also lower in potassium compared to other grains, making them a good choice for a CKD-friendly diet

If you have CKD and diabetes, it's best to eat carbs that are complex and don't raise your blood sugar quickly. Foods like whole grains, veggies, and beans are good choices. Try to avoid sugary foods and processed carbs because they can make your blood sugar go up fast.

2. Dietary Guidelines for CKD

Understanding the Renal Diet

Embarking on the journey through your renal diet means understanding and aligning your nutritional needs with your specific medical condition. The renal diet isn't a one-size-fits-all; it's a deeply personalized pathway that reflects your unique health circumstances and strives to support your kidney function effectively. This book underscores not merely what foods you should embrace or sidestep, but fundamentally seeks to empower you to adapt and shape your diet to mirror the specific needs of your condition.

Understanding that reducing protein intake or limiting phosphorus and potassium may not blanketly apply to every individual with CKD, this guide casts light on how to adaptively manage these elements. It will present as your companion in carving out a nourishing diet, always keeping the optimal functioning and health of your kidneys at the forefront.

It is absolutely normal to feel overwhelmed by all this amount of knowledge and responsibility!

This is not merely a book. It's a guide, a friend, and a resource, providing easy, delicious, and kidney-conscious recipes, which not only satisfy your taste buds but also adhere to the nutritional guidelines essential for your health. From understanding the basics of a renal diet to mastering the art of creating flavorful yet safe dishes, this book aims to reclaim a semblance of normalcy, freedom, and delight back into your meal times, ensuring you feel validated and embraced in every culinary choice you make.

Together, let's weave through the essential nutritional scaffolds vital for effective CKD management, demystifying how to sculpt a diet that's renal-friendly, personalized and testy.

Food to Embrace and Food to Avoid

Creating a comprehensive table of foods to eat and avoid for patients with chronic kidney disease is highly reductive as dietary needs can change significantly based on the stage of the disease, other health conditions, and dietary restrictions a person may have. However, here is a general guide that might be helpful. Please note that individual needs can vary widely and any changes in diet should be discussed with a healthcare professional.

Food Category	Embrace	Avoid or Limit	Notes
Fruits	Apples, Berries, Cherries, Grapes, Pineapple	Bananas, Oranges, Kiwi, Prunes, Avocados	Choose low-potassium fruits; limit intake of high-potassium fruits.
Vegetables	Cabbage, Green Beans, Bell Peppers, Zucchini	Potatoes, Tomatoes, Spinach, Swiss Chard	Opt for vegetables lower in potassium; be mindful of portion sizes for those that are higher.
Proteins	Lean cuts of Poultry, Fish, Tofu	Red Meats, Processed Meats, Nuts and Seeds	Ensure adequate protein without overconsuming; choose lean, low-sodium options where possible.
Dairy	Non-dairy alternatives (almond milk, rice milk)	Milk, Cheese, Yogurt	Limit phosphorus intake by choosing non-dairy alternatives when possible.
Grains	Rice, Buckwheat, Couscous	Whole-wheat Bread, Oatmeal	Refined grains are often lower in potassium and phosphorus compared to whole grains.
Snacks	Popcorn (unsalted), Rice Cakes	Chips, Nuts, Chocolate	Choose snacks low in sodium, potassium, and phosphorus; focus on portion control.
Drinks	Water, Clear Soda, Homemade Fruit Juices	Store-bought Fruit Juices, Alcohol, Coffee	Limit fluids if advised by healthcare provider; avoid high-potassium and high-phosphorus drinks.
Cereals	Cream of Rice, Cornflakes	Bran Cereals, Granola	Choose cereals that are lower in phosphorus and potassium.
Condiments	Fresh Herbs, Spices, Vinegar	Salt, Bouillon Cubes, Tomato Sauce	Use fresh herbs and spices to flavor food instead of salt; watch for hidden sodium in condiments.

Fluid: How to Stay Hydrated

Maintaining proper hydration in CKD patients is a delicate balance. While adequate fluid intake is vital for everyone, CKD patients may need to modulate this based on their individual renal functionality and doctor's guidelines. Fluid balance, crucial for managing waste and electrolyte regulation, can become disrupted as renal disease progresses. Individuals might experience either fluid retention, leading to swelling and high blood pressure, or struggle to conserve water, resulting in dehydration. For patients on dialysis, attentiveness to fluid intake becomes even more critical as extra consumption may pose challenges during the treatment. A personalized, doctor-advised fluid strategy ensures hydration without overburdening the kidneys.

Sources of Hydration for CKD Patients:
- Water: Always the top pick, albeit in regulated amounts as per medical advice.
- Low-Potassium Fruits: Like apples or pears, which are hydrating yet CKD-friendly.
- Vegetables: Opt for those with lower potassium, like cucumber and radishes.
- Herbal Teas: A potential choice, ensuring they're caffeine-free and suitable for renal diets.

Did you know that certain herbal teas, like chamomile or mint, can be not just hydrating but also potentially soothing for the renal system? However, ensuring they are decaffeinated and consulting with a healthcare provider are key steps to ensure they fit into your fluid strategy harmoniously.

3. Planning and Preparing Your Meals

Setting Up a Renal-Friendly Kitchen

A renal-friendly kitchen isn't merely about the foods it houses but also concerns the organization, accessibility, and presence of tools that facilitate kidney-conscious cooking and eating.

Organize Your Pantry: Maintain distinct sections for kidney-friendly items and those reserved for guests or other family members.

- **Kitchen Tools:** Ensure availability of measuring teacups, scales, and other tools for precise nutrient management.
- **Cookware:** Non-stick pans can aid in cooking with with minimal oil and facilitate easier cleanup. Consider pots and pans of various sizes for different preparation needs.
- **Spice Rack:** Cultivate a collection of spices and herbs to enhance flavor without leaning on sodium.
- **Accessible Healthy Snacks:** Designate a specific, easy-to-reach spot for kidney-friendly snacks like unsalted nuts or seeds.

Creating a conducive kitchen environment makes adhering to your renal diet both convenient and straightforward, thereby setting a seamless stage for kidney health nourishment.

Remember, an organized kitchen that distinctly separates renal-friendly components from others avoids accidental dietary missteps and eases the daily culinary process.

Reading Food Labels: Decoding Ingredient

Understanding food labels is akin to mastering a secret language that deciphers the pathway to kidney wellness. Accurate decoding of labels leads to empowered decisions, curating a diet that aligns with your renal health goals while avoiding the pitfall of hidden, harmful components.

The information not to be missed:
- **Serving Size:** Always check the serving size first. All the information on the label applies to this specific amount of food. If you eat more or less than the listed serving size, you'll need to adjust the values accordingly.
- **Daily Value:** You'll see "% Daily Value" on the label. This helps you understand whether the amount of sodium in one serving of the food is high or low. 5% DV or less is low, and 20% DV or more is high.
- **Amount of Sodium:** The sodium content will be listed in milligrams (mg). It's crucial to keep this in check, especially for individuals monitoring their sodium intake for health reasons.
- **Sodium-Free or Low-Sodium?:** Check if the product is labeled as "sodium-free" (less than 5mg per serving), "very low sodium" (35mg or less), or "low sodium" (140mg or less).
- **Other Nutrients:** Remember that sodium is not the only important factor. Make sure to check for other essential nutrients like potassium and phosphorus, particularly in the context of renal health.

Alternative terms that may be found in the food labels:

Term(s)	Nutrient	Notes for CKD Patients
Na, Sodium, Baking soda (sodium bicarbonate), MSG (monosodium glutamate)	Sodium	Keep intake within the recommended limits by your healthcare provider, often between 1500-2300 mg per day.
K, Potassium, KCl	Potassium	Potassium intake may need to be limited in later stages of CKD to avoid hyperkalemia.
Phos, Phosphate, Phosphorus	Phosphorus	Phosphorus levels should be monitored and managed in CKD patients to avoid bone and cardiovascular issues.
Protein, Pea Protein, etc.	Protein	Protein intake may need to be managed, especially in later stages of CKD to reduce kidney workload.
Calcium, Ca	Calcium	Calcium needs can vary, and it's crucial to balance it with phosphorus for bone health.
Sugar, Sucrose, Fructose	Sugars	May not be directly related to kidney health, but managing blood sugar levels is crucial, especially for diabetic patients
Trans fat, Saturated fat	Unhealthy Fats	Keeping heart health in check is vital for CKD patients; therefore, managing fat intake becomes crucial.

Do you know the Plate Method? It is a simple way to plan balanced meals that provide all necessary nutrients. Consider employing it: half the plate filled with vegetables, a quarter with lean protein, and a quarter with grains or starches.

4. 1900 Days-Renal Diet Recipes: Navigating Through Alternatives

Guide to Food Substitutes

Recipes, no matter how delicious they are, can become tiresome when repeated too frequently.

"Renal Diet Cookbook for Beginners" offers more than just kidney-friendly recipes; it provides a versatile guide to achieving an incredible 1900 days of varied meals, despite CKD dietary restrictions. By strategically swapping components, as suggested in the book's detailed tables, you can continually reinvent dishes, ensuring your meals remain exciting and nutritionally appropriate. This guide doesn't only facilitate adherence to sodium, potassium, and phosphorus limits but also turns meal preparation into a delightful culinary adventure, making managing CKD dietary requirements both simple and enjoyable.

Imagine enjoying a different dish every day for over five years, all while adhering to the dietary recommendations for managing CKD!

Food Category	Common Food	Alternatives	Notes
Proteins	Chicken (3.5oz)	Turkey (3.5oz) Tofu (3.5oz) Egg whites (3)	Prefer low-sodium options or use fresh meat; tofu is a plant protein option.
	Salmon (3.5oz)	Tuna (3.5oz) Catfish (3.5oz) Trout (3.5oz)	Monitor for potassium content and ensure appropriate portion sizes.
Fruits	Apple (1 medium)	Pear (1 medium) Peach (1 medium) Plums (2 small)	All relatively low in potassium; consider portion sizes.
	Blueberries (1 teacup)	Cranberries (1/2 teacup) Strawberries (1/2 teacup) Raspberries (1/2 teacup)	Verify portion sizes; generally low in potassium and phosphorus.
Vegetables	Green beans (1 teacup)	Wax beans (1/2 teacup) Snow peas (1/2 teacup) Asparagus (1 teacup)	Consider potassium content and leaching methods where appropriate.
	Cabbage (1 teacup)	Cauliflower (1 teacup) Iceberg lettuce (1 teacup) Red bell pepper (1 medium)	Varying potassium levels; adjust per dietary needs.
Dairy/Dairy Alternatives	Rice milk (1 teacup)	Almond milk (1 teacup) Cashew milk (1 teacup) Oat milk (1 teacup)	Choose unenriched versions when possible; monitor for added phosphates.
	Hard cheese (1oz)	Cream cheese (1oz) Brie cheese (1oz) Camembert (1oz)	Sodium can vary; ensure it fits within dietary sodium limits.
Grains/Cereals	White rice (1 teacup)	Couscous (1/2 teacup) White pasta (1/2 teacup) Bulgar wheat (1/2 teacup)	Prefer refined grains; monitor for added phosphates.
	White bread (1 slice)	Pita bread (1 small pita) Bagel (1/2 small) English muffin (1/2)	Always check for added phosphates on labels.
Snacks	Popcorn (1 teacup, air-popped)	Rice cakes (1 cake) Unsalted pretzels (1oz) Unsalted crackers (5)	Ensure low sodium and potassium; monitor portion sizes.
	Apple slices (1 medium apple)	Grapes (1/2 teacup) Pineapple (1/2 teacup) Watermelon (1/2 teacup)	Refreshing and can be low in potassium; verify portions.
Drinks	Water (1 teacup)	Herbal tea (1 teacup) Apple juice (1 teacup) Grape juice (1 teacup)	Herbal teas and juice require confirmation from a dietitian for safety.
	Lemonade (1 teacup, homemade)	Limeade (1 teacup, homemade) Cranberry juice (1 teacup, unsweetened) Pear juice (1 teacup)	Prefer freshly squeezed or without added sugars and additives.

Note: This table is meant to present as a guide. It's critical to consult with healthcare professionals to create a personalized meal plan that aligns with individual health needs, considering all nutrient restrictions and requirements. Always remember that actual nutrient content may vary, and reading food labels, as well as managing portion sizes, are vital practices in maintaining a balanced renal diet.

Guide to Salt Substitutes

Navigating through dietary salts and their substitutes becomes an essential part of everyday meal planning and preparation. Understanding what's available, their nutrient content, and how they interact with your meals helps in creating not only nutritious but also flavorful dishes. Let's delve into some popular salt substitutes and how you might incorporate them into your recipes while keeping kidney health in mind.

Herbs and Spices

Usage: Employ fresh or dried herbs and spices to include layers of flavors to your dishes without the **added sodium.**

Examples: Basil, parsley, thyme, rosemary, garlic, onion, paprika, and more.

Note: Be mindful of spice blends in stores; opt for those labeled "sodium-free."

Vinegars

Usage: Enhance flavors, particularly in soups and salads, with a splash of various vinegars.

Examples: Apple cider vinegar, balsamic vinegar, rice vinegar, etc.

Note: Ensure that the chosen vinegar complements the dish's flavor profile.

Lemon or Lime Juice

Usage: A dash of citrus can elevate flavors, especially in fish dishes, salads, and beverages.

Note: Citrus can also alter the taste of certain components, so include judiciously.

Seaweed Products

Usage: Seaweed granules or powders can include a distinct, oceanic flavor to dishes, mimicking a saltiness without actual sodium.

Note: Ensure they are low in sodium and potassium to be suitable for a renal diet.

Fennel Seeds

Usage: A mildly sweet and anise-like flavor, they can be used whole or ground in various dishes.

Note: Utilize them in moderation as they possess a potent flavor.

Celery Juice or Powder

Usage: Celery contains natural sodium but in lower amounts compared to table salt.

Note: Be mindful of the amount used and monitor its impact on overall sodium intake.

Hing (Asafoetida)

Usage: Used widely in Indian cooking, it provides a savory, umami-like flavor, especially good for lentil dishes.

Note: Ensure to use pure hing, as some commercially available variants may have added salt.

Za'atar

Usage: A Middle Eastern spice blend involving sesame seeds, sumac, and herbs that include a robust, tangy flavor.

Note: Opt for homemade blends where you can control the sodium content.

Tamarind Paste

Usage: Provides a sour and mildly sweet flavor, commonly utilized in Asian and Indian cuisines.

Note: Look for versions with no added salts and utilize in moderation.

Carob Powder

Usage: Can provide a naturally sweet flavor, often used as a cocoa alternative but can also be utilized to balance savory dishes.

Note: Ensure it is pure carob powder without added sugars or salts.

Mushroom Powder

Usage: Ground dried mushrooms can lend an earthy, umami flavor to dishes, providing depth without salt.

Note: Use sparingly and monitor for any additional dietary implications.

Black Garlic

    Usage: Fermented garlic that adds a sweet, savory flavor to dishes, useful in various cuisines.

    Note: Be mindful of its potent flavor, ensuring it complements the dish.

Capers

    Usage: Provide a tangy, briny flavor. Use them fresh or look for versions preserved without salt.

    Note: Due to their briny nature, they should be used cautiously and sparingly

Considerations in Using Alternatives

    Taste and Adjust: Experimenting with these alternatives may require some taste testing and adjusting to hit the right note.

    Know Your Limits: Understanding your dietary restrictions, particularly concerning sodium, potassium, and phosphorus, is crucial.

    Embrace Experimentation: Engage in culinary explorations, trying different alternatives, and discovering new flavor profiles.

Remember: Consulting a healthcare professional or dietitian prior to introducing new elements to a renal diet is crucial to manage and optimize kidney health while relishing a range of flavorful foods.

Breakfast
Recipes

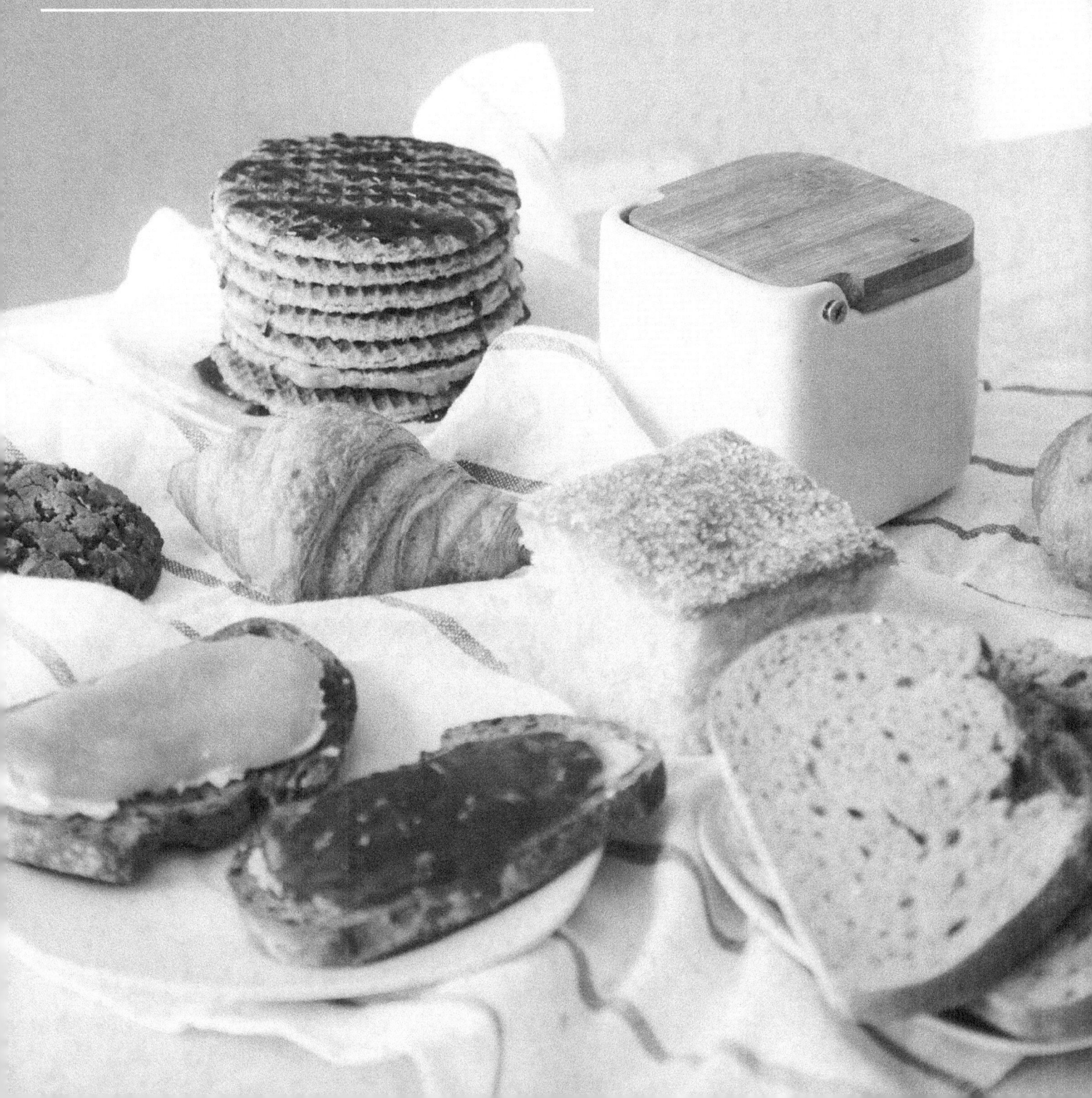

01 Apple Cinnamon Quinoa Porridge

Ingredients

Preparation time	Cooking time	Servings
5 MIN	15 MIN	2

- 1/2 teacup quinoa, washed and drained
- 1 teacup unsweetened applesauce
- 1/2 tsp ground cinnamon
- 1/2 teacupcubed apple (without the skin)
- 1 tbsp honey (elective, for sweetness)

Per serving:
Calories: 250kcal;
Fat: 2g;
Carbs: 56g;
Protein: 5g;
Sodium: 5mg;
Potassium: 225mg;
Phosphorus: 120mg

Direction

1. Inside your small saucepan, blend quinoa, applesauce, and ground cinnamon.
2. Boil, then decrease temp. to low, cover, then simmer for 12-15 mins or 'til quinoa is soft then has immersed most of the liquid.
3. Stir in cubed apple then cook for an extra 2-3 mins.
4. Sweeten with honey if anticipated.
5. Present warm.

02 Blueberry Rice Pancakes

Ingredients

PREPARATION TIME	COOKING TIME	SERVINGS
10 MIN	10 MIN	2

- 1 teacup cooked white rice (cooled)
- 1/2 teacup blueberries (fresh or frozen)
- 1/2 tsp vanilla extract
- 1/4 tsp ground cinnamon
- 2 eggs

Per serving:
Calories: 235kcal;
Fat: 6g;
Carbs: 37g;
Protein: 8g;
Sodium: 120mg;
Potassium: 120mg;
Phosphorus: 150mg

Direction

1. Inside your container, blend collectively cooked rice, blueberries, vanilla extract, and ground cinnamon.
2. Inside your distinct container, beat the eggs and then include them to the rice solution.
3. Warm yournon-stick griddle in a middling temp and mildlyoil it.
4. Pour your rice solution onto your griddle to form pancakes.
5. Cook for 3-4 mins on all sides or 'til golden brown.
6. Present hot.

0 3 Vegetable Scrambled Eggs

Ingredients

PREPARATION TIME · COOKING TIME · SERVINGS
5 MIN · 10 MIN · 2

- 4 big eggs
- 1/4 teacup cubed bell peppers
- 1/4 teacup cubed onions
- 1/4 teacup cubed zucchini
- 1/4 teacup cubed mushrooms
- Salt and pepper as needed

Per serving:
Calories: 150kcal;
Fat: 10g;
Carbs: 5g;
Protein: 12g;
Sodium: 140mg;
Potassium: 200mg;
Phosphorus: 150mg

Direction

1. Inside yournon-stick griddle, sauté the cubed vegetables in a middling temptill they become soft (around 5mins).
2. Inside your container, whisk the eggs and flavour using salt and pepper.
3. Pour your eggs over the sautéed vegetables and scramble tillthoroughly cooked.
4. Present hot.

0 4 Rice Flour Waffles with Fresh Berries

Ingredients

PREPARATION TIME · COOKING TIME · SERVINGS
10 MIN · 10 MIN · 2

- 1 teacup rice flour
- 1 tsp baking powder
- 1/2 teacup unsweetened almond milk
- 1/4 tsp vanilla extract
- Fresh mixed berries for topping (blueberries, strawberries, raspberries)

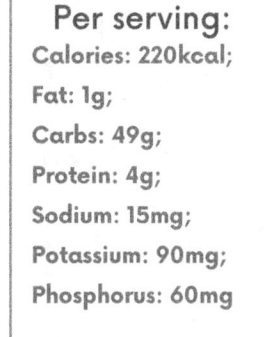

Per serving:
Calories: 220kcal;
Fat: 1g;
Carbs: 49g;
Protein: 4g;
Sodium: 15mg;
Potassium: 90mg;
Phosphorus: 60mg

Direction

1. Warm up your waffle iron using the manufacturer's guidelines.
2. Inside your container, whisk collectively rice flour, baking powder, almond milk, and vanilla extract till you have a smooth batter.
3. Pour your batter onto your warmed up waffle iron then cook till golden brown.
4. Top with fresh mixed berries.

0 5 Pineapple Mint Smoothie

Ingredients

PREPARATION TIME **5** MIN COOKING TIME **0** MIN SERVINGS **2**

- 1 teacup fresh or tinned pineapple chunks (unsweetened)
- 1/2 teacup fresh spinach leaves
- 1/2 teacup plain Greek yogurt
- 1/2 teacup water
- 1 tbsp fresh mint leaves
- Ice cubes (elective)

Per serving:
Calories: 120kcal;
Fat: 1g;
Carbs: 20g;
Protein: 7g;
Sodium: 60mg;
Potassium: 250mg;
Phosphorus: 75mg

Direction

1. Put the entirecomponentsinside a mixer.
2. Blend 'til smooth and creamy.
3. Put ice cubes if anticipated for a colder smoothie.
4. Pour into glasses and present.

0 6 Cucumber and Egg Breakfast Wrap

Ingredients

PREPARATION TIME **10** MIN COOKING TIME **5** MIN SERVINGS **2**

- 2 big eggs
- 1/4 teacupcubed cucumber
- 1 tbspcubed red bell pepper
- 1 tbspcubed green bell pepper
- Salt and pepper as needed
- 2 whole wheat or low-sodium tortillas

Per serving:
Calories: 180kcal;
Fat: 7g;
Carbs: 19g;
Protein: 11g;
Sodium: 200mg;
Potassium: 200mg;
Phosphorus: 120mg

Direction

1. Inside your container, whisk the eggs and flavour using salt and pepper.
2. Warm yournon-stick griddle inside a middling temp and mildlyoil it.
3. Pour your whisked eggs into your griddle and include the cubed vegetables.
4. Scramble the eggs tillthoroughly cooked.
5. Warm the tortillas in your microwave for a couple ofsecs.
6. Spoon your egg solution onto your tortillas and roll them up.
7. Present warm.

0 7 Carrot and Zucchini Muffins

Ingredients

PREPARATION TIME **15** MIN   COOKING TIME **20** MIN   SERVINGS **12**

- 1 teacup grated carrots
- 1 teacup grated zucchini
- 2 teacups whole wheat flour
- 1/2 teacup unsweetened applesauce
- 1/4 teacup honey
- 2 big eggs
- 1 tsp baking powder
- 1/2 tsp ground cinnamon

Per serving:
Calories: 120kcal;
Fat: 1g;
Carbs: 26g;
Protein: 3g;
Sodium: 60mg;
Potassium: 150mg;
Phosphorus: 90mg

Direction

1. Warm up your oven to 350 deg. F then line your muffin tin using paper liners.
2. Inside your container, blend baking powder, grated carrots, grated zucchini, whole wheat flour, and ground cinnamon.
3. Inside your extra container, whisk collectively applesauce, honey, and eggs.
4. Put your wet components into your dry components and mix till well blended.
5. Spoon your batter into your muffin tin, filling each teacuparound 2/3 full.
6. Bake for 20-25 mins or 'til a muffin when probed with a toothpick, the end result should be clean.
7. Allow the muffins to cool prior to serving.

0 8 Rice Cereal with Sliced Pears

Ingredients

PREPARATION TIME **5** MIN   COOKING TIME **5** MIN   SERVINGS **2**

- 1 teacup cooked white rice
- 1 ripe pear, finelycarved
- 1/4 tsp ground cinnamon
- 1/4 teacup unsweetened almond milk
- 1 tbsp honey (elective)

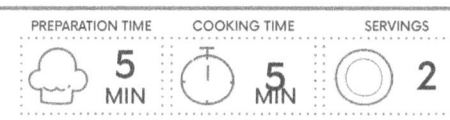

Per serving:
Calories: 180kcal;
Fat: 1g;
Carbs: 43g;
Protein: 2g;
Sodium: 5mg;
Potassium: 160mg;
Phosphorus: 70mg

Direction

1. Inside your saucepot, blend cooked rice, carved pear, ground cinnamon, and almond milk.
2. Heat at low-middling temp, mixing irregularlytill fully heated and pear is soft (around 5mins).
3. Sweeten with honey if anticipated.
4. Present warm.

0 9 Peach Yogurt Parfait

Ingredients

PREPARATION TIME **5** MIN | COOKING TIME **0** MIN | SERVINGS **2**

- 1 teacup non-dairy yogurt (like almond or soy yogurt)
- 1 teacuptinned peaches (with its own juice), drained and cubed
- 1/4 teacup granola (low-sodium and low-phosphorus)
- 1 tbsp honey (elective)

Per serving:
Calories: 220kcal;
Fat: 4g;
Carbs: 42g;
Protein: 4g;
Sodium: 20mg;
Potassium: 250mg;
Phosphorus: 100mg

Direction

1. In two serving glasses or containers, layer non-dairy yogurt, cubed peaches, and granola.
2. Spray with honey for sweetness if anticipated.
3. Repeat the layers.
4. Present chilled.

1 0 Veggie Omelet with Fresh Herbs

Ingredients

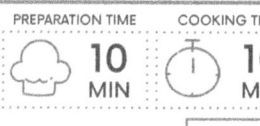 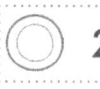

PREPARATION TIME **10** MIN | COOKING TIME **10** MIN | SERVINGS **2**

- 4 big eggs
- 1/4 teacupcubed bell peppers
- 1/4 teacupcubed onions
- 1/4 teacupcubed zucchini
- 1/4 teacupcubed mushrooms
- Fresh herbs (like parsley or chives)
- Salt and pepper as needed

Per serving:
Calories: 160kcal;
Fat: 10g;
Carbs: 7g;
Protein: 12g;
Sodium: 120mg;
Potassium: 250mg;
Phosphorus: 150mg

Direction

1. Inside your container, whisk the eggs and flavour using salt and pepper.
2. Warm yournon-stick griddle in a middling temp and mildlyoil it.
3. Pour your whisked eggs into your griddle and include the cubed vegetables.
4. Cook till the edges start to set, then spray fresh herbs on one half of the omelet.
5. Wrap the other half of the omelet over the herbs then cook till fully set.
6. Slide the omelet onto a plate then garnish with additional fresh herbs.
7. Present hot.

11 Cauliflower Breakfast Hash

Ingredients

PREPARATION TIME 10 MIN COOKING TIME 15 MIN SERVINGS 2

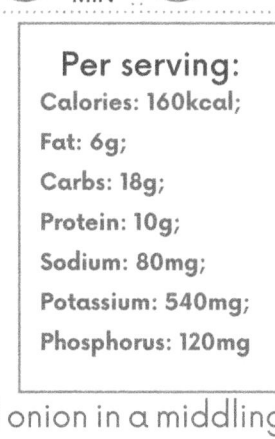

- 2 teacups cauliflower florets, severed
- 1/2 teacupcubed red bell pepper
- 1/2 teacupcubed onion
- 2 big eggs
- 1/4 tsp garlic powder
- Salt and pepper as needed
- Fresh parsley for garnish (elective)

Per serving:
Calories: 160kcal;
Fat: 6g;
Carbs: 18g;
Protein: 10g;
Sodium: 80mg;
Potassium: 540mg;
Phosphorus: 120mg

Direction

1. Inside yournon-stick griddle, sauté the cauliflower, red bell pepper, and onion in a middling temptill they become soft (around 10mins).
2. Make two wells in your cauliflower solution and crack the eggs into each well.
3. Spray with garlic powder, salt, and pepper.
4. Cover then cook for around 5mins or 'til the eggs are cooked to your wants.
5. Garnish using fresh parsley if anticipated.
6. Present hot.

12 Raspberry Almond Breakfast Quinoa

Ingredients

PREPARATION TIME 5 MIN COOKING TIME 15 MIN SERVINGS 2

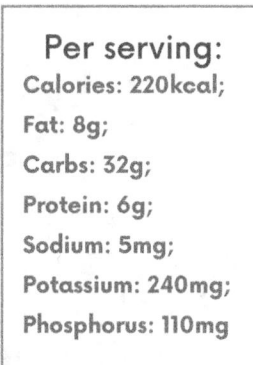

- 1 teacup cooked quinoa
- 1/2 teacup fresh raspberries
- 1/4 teacupcarved almonds (use sparingly for lower phosphorus)
- 1/2 tsp almond extract
- 1 tbsp honey (elective)

Per serving:
Calories: 220kcal;
Fat: 8g;
Carbs: 32g;
Protein: 6g;
Sodium: 5mg;
Potassium: 240mg;
Phosphorus: 110mg

Direction

1. Inside your container, blend cooked quinoa, fresh raspberries, and carved almonds.
2. Include almond extract and mix well.
3. Sweeten with honey if anticipated.
4. Present warm.

13 Sautéed Mushroom and Onion Frittata

Ingredients

PREPARATION TIME 10 MIN   COOKING TIME 15 MIN   SERVINGS 2

- 4 big eggs
- 1 teacupcarved mushrooms
- 1/2 teacupcubed onion
- 1/4 teacup grated Parmesan cheese
- Salt and pepper as needed

Per serving:
Calories: 210kcal;
Fat: 14g;
Carbs: 7g;
Protein: 14g;
Sodium: 250mg;
Potassium: 340mg;
Phosphorus: 210mg

Direction

1. Inside your container, whisk the eggs and flavour using salt and pepper.
2. Warm yournon-stick griddle in a middling temp and mildlyoil it.
3. Includecarved mushrooms and cubed onion to the griddle and sauté tillsoft (around 5mins).
4. Pour your whisked eggs over the vegetables and spray with grated Parmesan cheese.
5. Cook for around 5-7 mins or 'til the edges are set.
6. Transfer the griddle to a warmed up broiler and broil for 2-3 mins 'til the top is golden brown.
7. Slice into wedges and present.

14 Lemon and Blueberry Rice Cakes

Ingredients

PREPARATION TIME 5 MIN   COOKING TIME 0 MIN   SERVINGS 2

- 2 rice cakes (low-sodium)
- 1/2 teacup fresh blueberries
- Zest of 1 lemon
- 2 tbsps lemon juice
- 1 tbsp honey (elective)

Per serving:
Calories: 70kcal;
Fat: 0g;
Carbs: 18g;
Protein: 1g;
Sodium: 0mg;
Potassium: 40mg;
Phosphorus: 20mg

Direction

1. Put your rice cakes on your serving plate.
2. Inside your container, blend collectively fresh blueberries, lemon zest, and lemon juice.
3. Spoon your blueberry solution onto your rice cakes.
4. Spray with honey for sweetness if anticipated.
5. Presentinstantly.

1 5 Fresh Berry and Rice Milk Smoothie

PREPARATION TIME 5 MIN COOKING TIME 0 MIN SERVINGS 2

Ingredients

- 1 teacup unsweetened rice milk
- 1 teacup mixed fresh berries (e.g., strawberries, blueberries, raspberries)
- 1/2 banana
- 1/2 tsp vanilla extract
- Ice cubes (elective)

Per serving:
Calories: 70kcal;
Fat: 0g;
Carbs: 17g;
Protein: 1g;
Sodium: 60mg;
Potassium: 220mg;
Phosphorus: 100mg

Direction

1. Put the entirecomponentsinside a mixer.
2. Blend 'til smooth and creamy.
3. Put ice cubes if anticipated for a colder smoothie.
4. Pour into glasses and present.

1 6 Pear and Cinnamon Breakfast Rice

Ingredients

PREPARATION TIME 10 MIN COOKING TIME 20 MIN SERVINGS 2

- 1 teacup cooked white rice
- 1 ripe pear, cubed
- 1/2 tsp ground cinnamon
- 1/4 teacup unsweetened almond milk
- 1 tbsp honey (elective)

Per serving:
Calories: 190kcal;
Fat: 1g;
Carbs: 45g;
Protein: 2g;
Sodium: 10mg;
Potassium: 170mg;
Phosphorus: 75mg

Direction

1. Inside your saucepot, blend cooked rice, cubed pear, ground cinnamon, and almond milk.
2. Heat at low-middling temp, mixing irregularlytill fully heated and pear is soft (around 10mins).
3. Sweeten with honey if anticipated.
4. Present warm.

17 Spinach and Egg White Scramble

PREPARATION TIME	COOKING TIME	SERVINGS
5 MIN	5 MIN	2

Ingredients

- 4 big egg whites
- 1 teacup fresh spinach leaves
- 1/4 teacupcubed onion
- Salt and pepper as needed

Per serving:
Calories: 40kcal;
Fat: 0g;
Carbs: 3g;
Protein: 8g;
Sodium: 95mg;
Potassium: 210mg;
Phosphorus: 50mg

Direction

1. Inside your container, whisk the egg whites and flavour using salt and pepper.
2. Warm yournon-stick griddle in a middling temp and mildlyoil it.
3. Includecubed onion and spinach to the griddle and sauté till the spinach wilts (around 2-3 mins).
4. Pour your whisked egg whites over the vegetables and scramble tillthoroughly cooked.
5. Present hot.

18 Pineapple and Coconut Chia Pudding

PREPARATION TIME	COOKING TIME	SERVINGS
10 MIN	0 MIN	2

Ingredients

- 1/4 teacup chia seeds
- 1 teacup unsweetened coconut milk
- 1/2 teacupcubed pineapple (fresh or tinned in its own juice)
- 1 tbspteared up coconut (unsweetened)
- 1 tbsp honey (elective)

Per serving:
Calories: 180kcal;
Fat: 10g;
Carbs: 21g;
Protein: 4g;
Sodium: 30mg;
Potassium: 140mg;
Phosphorus: 120mg

Direction

1. Inside your container, mix chia seeds and coconut milk. Stir well and allow it to relax for 5 mins.
2. Stir again to prevent clumping, cover, then put in the fridge for almost 2 hrs or overnight till it thickens.
3. Before serving, top with cubed pineapple, teared up coconut, and spray with honey if anticipated.
4. Present chilled.

19 Warm Millet Bowl with Fresh Berries

Ingredients

PREPARATION TIME 10 MIN
COOKING TIME 20 MIN
SERVINGS 2

- 1/2 teacup dry millet
- 1 teacup water
- 1/2 teacup mixed fresh berries (e.g., strawberries, blueberries, raspberries)
- 1/4 tsp ground cinnamon
- 1/4 teacup unsweetened almond milk
- 1 tbsp honey (elective)

Per serving:
Calories: 230kcal;
Fat: 2g;
Carbs: 48g;
Protein: 5g;
Sodium: 5mg;
Potassium: 190mg;
Phosphorus: 120mg

Direction

1. Rinse millet under cold water and drain.
2. Inside your saucepot, blend millet and water. Boil, then decrease temp., cover, then simmer for 15-20 mins 'til millet is soft and water is immersed.
3. Fluff the cooked millet using a fork and stir in ground cinnamon.
4. Spoon into serving containers then top with fresh berries.
5. Spray with almond milk and honey if anticipated.
6. Present warm.

20 Rice and Almond Breakfast Pudding

Ingredients

PREPARATION TIME 10 MIN
COOKING TIME 0 MIN
SERVINGS 2

- 1 teacup cooked white rice
- 1/4 teacup unsweetened almond milk
- 1/4 tsp almond extract
- 1/4 teacupcarved almonds (use sparingly for lower phosphorus)
- 1 tbsp honey (elective)

Per serving:
Calories: 220kcal;
Fat: 8g;
Carbs: 34g;
Protein: 4g;
Sodium: 5mg;
Potassium: 70mg;
Phosphorus: 45mg

Direction

1. Inside your container, mix cooked rice, almond milk, and almond extract.
2. Stir well and allow it to relax in your fridge for almost 1 hr or 'til chilled.
3. Before serving, top with carved almonds and spray with honey if anticipated.
4. Present cold.

Soup
Recipes

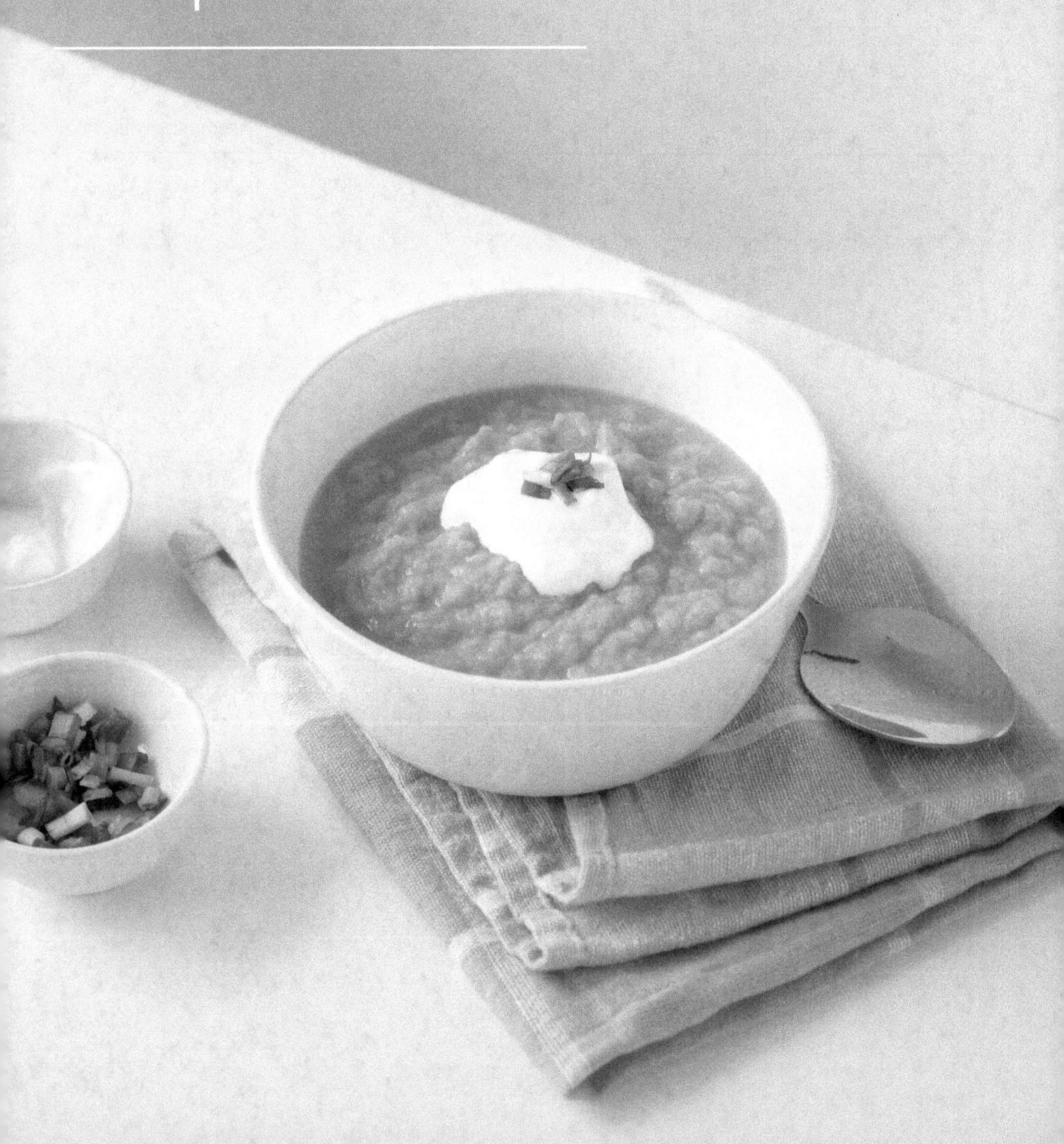

2 1 Carrot and Ginger Soup

Ingredients

PREPARATION TIME	COOKING TIME	SERVINGS
10 MIN	20 MIN	4

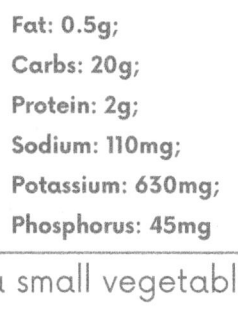

- 4 teacups low-sodium vegetable broth
- 4 teacupssevered carrots
- 1 small onion, cubed
- 1-inch piece of ginger, skinned and crushed
- 1/2 tsp ground black pepper
- 1/2 tsp dried thyme
- 1/2 tsp garlic powder

Per serving:
Calories: 85kcal;
Fat: 0.5g;
Carbs: 20g;
Protein: 2g;
Sodium: 110mg;
Potassium: 630mg;
Phosphorus: 45mg

Direction

1. Inside your big pot, sauté the cubed onion and crushed ginger inside a small vegetable broth till softened.
2. Include the severed carrots, thyme, garlic powder, and black pepper. Cook for a couple of more mins.
3. Pour in your vegetable broth then boil. Decrease temp., cover, then simmer till the carrots are soft (around 15-20 mins).
4. Use immersion mixer to puree the soup 'til smooth.
5. Present hot.

2 2 Chicken and Rice Soup

Ingredients

PREPARATION TIME	COOKING TIME	SERVINGS
10 MIN	25 MIN	4

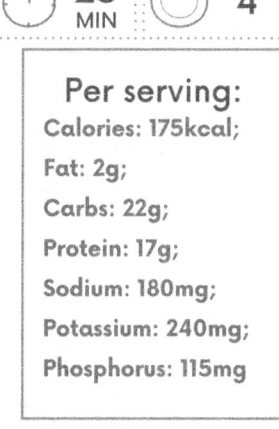

- 4 teacups low-sodium chicken broth
- 1 teacup cooked chicken breast, teared up
- 1 teacup cooked white rice
- 1 teacup carrots, cubed
- 1/2 teacup celery, cubed
- 1/2 tsp dried thyme
- 1/2 tsp garlic powder
- Salt and pepper as needed

Per serving:
Calories: 175kcal;
Fat: 2g;
Carbs: 22g;
Protein: 17g;
Sodium: 180mg;
Potassium: 240mg;
Phosphorus: 115mg

Direction

1. Inside your big pot, blend chicken broth, carrots, celery, thyme, and garlic powder.
2. Boil, then decrease temp. then simmer till the vegetables are soft (around 15-20 mins).
3. Include the cooked chicken and rice. Simmer for an extra 5 mins.
4. Flavour using salt and pepper as needed.
5. Present hot.

2 3 Butternut Squash Soup

Ingredients

	PREPARATION TIME	COOKING TIME	SERVINGS
	10 MIN	30 MIN	4

- 4 teacups low-sodium vegetable broth
- 4 teacupsskinned and cubed butternut squash
- 1 small onion, cubed
- 1/2 tsp ground nutmeg
- 1/2 tsp ground cinnamon
- Salt and pepper as needed

Per serving:
Calories: 85kcal;
Fat: 0.5g;
Carbs: 22g;
Protein: 1g;
Sodium: 150mg;
Potassium: 440mg;
Phosphorus: 30mg

Direction

1. Inside your big pot, blend vegetable broth, butternut squash, and cubed onion.
2. Boil, then decrease temp. then simmer till the squash is soft (around 20-25 mins).
3. Use immersion mixer to puree the soup 'til smooth.
4. Stir in nutmeg and cinnamon. Flavour using salt and pepper.
5. Present hot.

2 4 Cauliflower and Leek Soup

Ingredients

	PREPARATION TIME	COOKING TIME	SERVINGS
	10 MIN	20 MIN	4

- 4 teacups low-sodium vegetable broth
- 4 teacups cauliflower florets
- 2 leeks, white & light green parts only, severed
- 1/2 tsp dried thyme
- 1/2 tsp garlic powder
- Salt and pepper as needed

Per serving:
Calories: 45kcal;
Fat: 0.5g;
Carbs: 10g;
Protein: 2g;
Sodium: 170mg;
Potassium: 370mg;
Phosphorus: 45mg

Direction

1. Inside your big pot, blend vegetable broth, cauliflower florets, severed leeks, thyme, and garlic powder.
2. Boil, then decrease temp. then simmer till the cauliflower is soft (around 20-25 mins).
3. Use immersion mixer to puree the soup 'til smooth.
4. Flavour using salt and pepper as needed.
5. Present hot.

2 5 Celery and Green Apple Soup

Ingredients

PREPARATION TIME 10 MIN
COOKING TIME 25 MIN
SERVINGS 4

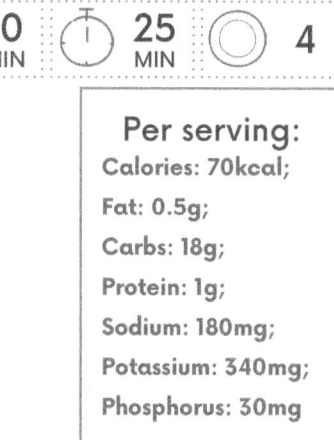

- 4 teacups low-sodium vegetable broth
- 4 teacups celery, severed
- 2 green apples, skinned, cored, and severed
- 1/2 tsp dried thyme
- 1/2 tsp garlic powder
- Salt and pepper as needed

Per serving:
Calories: 70kcal;
Fat: 0.5g;
Carbs: 18g;
Protein: 1g;
Sodium: 180mg;
Potassium: 340mg;
Phosphorus: 30mg

Direction

1. Inside your big pot, blend vegetable broth, severed celery, severed green apples, thyme, and garlic powder.
2. Boil, then decrease temp. then simmer till the celery and apples are soft (around 20-25 mins).
3. Use immersion mixer to puree the soup 'til smooth.
4. Flavour using salt and pepper as needed.
5. Present hot.

2 6 Simple Vegetable Broth Soup

Ingredients

PREPARATION TIME 10 MIN
COOKING TIME 20 MIN
SERVINGS 4

- 4 teacups low-sodium vegetable broth
- 2 teacups mixed vegetables (e.g., carrots, celery, green beans), severed
- 1 small onion, cubed
- 1/2 tsp dried thyme
- 1/2 tsp garlic powder
- Salt and pepper as needed

Per serving:
Calories: 40kcal;
Fat: 0.2g;
Carbs: 9g;
Protein: 1g;
Sodium: 100mg;
Potassium: 200mg;
Phosphorus: 25mg

Direction

1. Inside your big pot, blend vegetable broth, mixed vegetables, cubed onion, thyme, and garlic powder.
2. Boil, then decrease temp. then simmer till the vegetables are soft (around 15-20 mins).
3. Flavour using salt and pepper as needed.
4. Present hot.

27 Pumpkin and Sage Soup

PREPARATION TIME	COOKING TIME	SERVINGS
10 MIN	30 MIN	4

Ingredients

- 4 teacups low-sodium vegetable broth
- 2 teacupstinned pumpkin puree (unsalted)
- 1 small onion, cubed
- 1 tsp dried sage
- 1/2 tsp ground nutmeg
- Salt and pepper as needed

Per serving:
Calories: 60kcal;
Fat: 0.5g;
Carbs: 15g;
Protein: 1g;
Sodium: 120mg;
Potassium: 380mg;
Phosphorus: 30mg

Direction

1. Inside your big pot, blend vegetable broth, pumpkin puree, cubed onion, sage, and nutmeg.
2. Boil, then decrease temp. then simmer for around 20-25 mins.
3. Flavour using salt and pepper as needed.
4. Present hot.

28 Cucumber and Dill Cold Soup

PREPARATION TIME	COOKING TIME	SERVINGS
10 MIN	0 MIN	4

Ingredients

- 2 cucumbers, skinned and cubed
- 2 teacups low-sodium vegetable broth
- 1 teacup plain Greek yogurt
- 2 tbsp fresh dill, severed
- 1 piece garlic, crushed
- Salt and pepper as needed

Per serving:
Calories: 60kcal;
Fat: 1g;
Carbs: 7g;
Protein: 6g;
Sodium: 80mg;
Potassium: 280mg;
Phosphorus: 70mg

Direction

1. Inside a mixer, blendcubed cucumbers, vegetable broth, Greek yogurt, fresh dill, and crushed garlic. Blend 'til smooth.
2. Chill the soup in your fridge for almost 1 hr prior to serving.
3. Flavour using salt and pepper as needed.
4. Present cold.

2 9 Zucchini and Yellow Squash Soup

Ingredients

PREPARATION TIME **10 MIN** COOKING TIME **25 MIN** SERVINGS **4**

- 4 teacups low-sodium vegetable broth
- 2 zucchinis, cubed
- 2 yellow squashes, cubed
- 1 small onion, cubed
- 1/2 tsp dried basil
- 1/2 tsp dried oregano
- Salt and pepper as needed

Per serving:
Calories: 50kcal;
Fat: 0.5g;
Carbs: 11g;
Protein: 2g;
Sodium: 120mg;
Potassium: 380mg;
Phosphorus: 45mg

Direction

1. Inside your big pot, blend vegetable broth, cubed zucchinis, cubed yellow squashes, cubed onion, basil, and oregano.
2. Boil, then decrease temp. then simmer till the vegetables are soft (around 20-25 mins).
3. Flavour using salt and pepper as needed.
4. Present hot.

3 0 White Fish and Veggie Soup

Ingredients

PREPARATION TIME **10 MIN** COOKING TIME **20 MIN** SERVINGS **4**

- 4 teacups low-sodium fish or vegetable broth
- 1 teacup white fish fillets (e.g., cod or tilapia), cubed
- 2 teacups mixed vegetables (e.g., carrots, broccoli, bell peppers), severed
- 1 small onion, cubed
- 1/2 tsp dried thyme
- 1/2 tsp garlic powder
- Salt and pepper as needed

Per serving:
Calories: 85kcal;
Fat: 0.5g;
Carbs: 9g;
Protein: 14g;
Sodium: 140mg;
Potassium: 350mg;
Phosphorus: 130mg

Direction

1. Inside your big pot, blend fish or vegetable broth, cubed white fish, mixed vegetables, cubed onion, thyme, and garlic powder.
2. Boil, then decrease temp. then simmer till the fish is thoroughly cooked then the vegetables are soft (around 15-20 mins).
3. Flavour using salt and pepper as needed.
4. Present hot.

3 1 Turkey and Wild Rice Soup

PREPARATION TIME 10 MIN — COOKING TIME 30 MIN — SERVINGS 4

Ingredients

- 4 teacups low-sodium chicken broth
- 2 teacups cooked turkey breast, cubed
- 1/2 teacup wild rice, cooked
- 1 teacup carrots, cubed
- 1/2 teacup celery, cubed
- 1 small onion, cubed
- 1/2 tsp dried thyme
- 1/2 tsp garlic powder
- Salt and pepper as needed

Per serving:
Calories: 180kcal;
Fat: 1.5g;
Carbs: 21g;
Protein: 20g;
Sodium: 150mg;
Potassium: 260mg;
Phosphorus: 175mg

Direction

1. Inside your big pot, blend chicken broth, cubed turkey breast, cooked wild rice, cubed carrots, cubed celery, cubed onion, thyme, and garlic powder.

2. Boil, then decrease temp. then simmer for around 20-25 mins.

3. Flavour using salt and pepper as needed.

4. Present hot

3 2 Lemon and Coriander Soup

PREPARATION TIME 10 MIN — COOKING TIME 20 MIN — SERVINGS 4

Ingredients

- 4 teacups low-sodium vegetable broth
- 2 lemons, juice and zest
- 1/2 teacup fresh coriander (cilantro), severed
- 1 small onion, cubed
- 1/2 tsp ground cumin
- 1/2 tsp ground coriander
- Salt and pepper as needed

Per serving:
Calories: 40kcal;
Fat: 0.5g;
Carbs: 9g;
Protein: 1g;
Sodium: 70mg;
Potassium: 130mg;
Phosphorus: 25mg

Direction

1. Inside your big pot, blend vegetable broth, lemon juice, lemon zest, severed fresh coriander, cubed onion, ground cumin, and ground coriander.

2. Boil, then decrease temp. then simmer for around 15-20 mins.

3. Flavour using salt and pepper as needed.

4. Present hot.

3 3 Roasted Red Pepper Soup

Ingredients

PREPARATION TIME 10 MIN COOKING TIME 25 MIN SERVINGS 4

- 4 teacups low-sodium vegetable broth
- 2 roasted red peppers, skinned and cubed (you can use jarred ones)
- 1 small onion, cubed
- 2 pieces garlic, crushed
- 1/2 tsp dried basil
- 1/2 tsp dried oregano
- Salt and pepper as needed

Per serving:
Calories: 30kcal;
Fat: 0g;
Carbs: 7g;
Protein: 1g;
Sodium: 90mg;
Potassium: 190mg;
Phosphorus: 20mg

Direction

1. Inside your big pot, blend vegetable broth, cubed roasted red peppers, cubed onion, crushed garlic, dried basil, and dried oregano.

2. Boil, then decrease temp. then simmer for around 20-25 mins.

3. Flavour using salt and pepper as needed.

4. Present hot.

3 4 Mushroom and Thyme Soup

Ingredients

PREPARATION TIME 10 MIN COOKING TIME 25 MIN SERVINGS 4

- 4 teacups low-sodium vegetable broth
- 2 teacups mushrooms, carved
- 1 small onion, cubed
- 2 pieces garlic, crushed
- 1/2 tsp dried thyme
- 1/2 tsp dried rosemary
- Salt and pepper as needed

Per serving:
Calories: 35kcal;
Fat: 0g;
Carbs: 6g;
Protein: 2g;
Sodium: 120mg;
Potassium: 230mg;
Phosphorus: 45mg

Direction

1. Inside your big pot, blend vegetable broth, carved mushrooms, cubed onion, crushed garlic, dried thyme, and dried rosemary.

2. Boil, then decrease temp. then simmer for around 20-25 mins.

3. Flavour using salt and pepper as needed.

4. Present hot.

3 5 Saffron and Cauliflower Soup

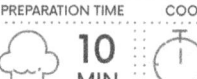 10 MIN   25 MIN   4

Ingredients

- 4 teacups low-sodium vegetable broth
- 4 teacups cauliflower florets
- 1 small onion, cubed
- 1/4 tsp saffron threads (elective)
- 1/2 tsp ground turmeric
- Salt and pepper as needed

Per serving:
Calories: 30kcal;
Fat: 0g;
Carbs: 7g;
Protein: 2g;
Sodium: 110mg;
Potassium: 370mg;
Phosphorus: 45mg

Direction

1. Inside your big pot, blend vegetable broth, cauliflower florets, cubed onion, saffron threads (if using), and ground turmeric.

2. Boil, then decrease temp. then simmer for around 20-25 mins.

3. Use immersion mixer to puree the soup 'til smooth.

4. Flavour using salt and pepper as needed.

5. Present hot.

Vegetarian

Recipes

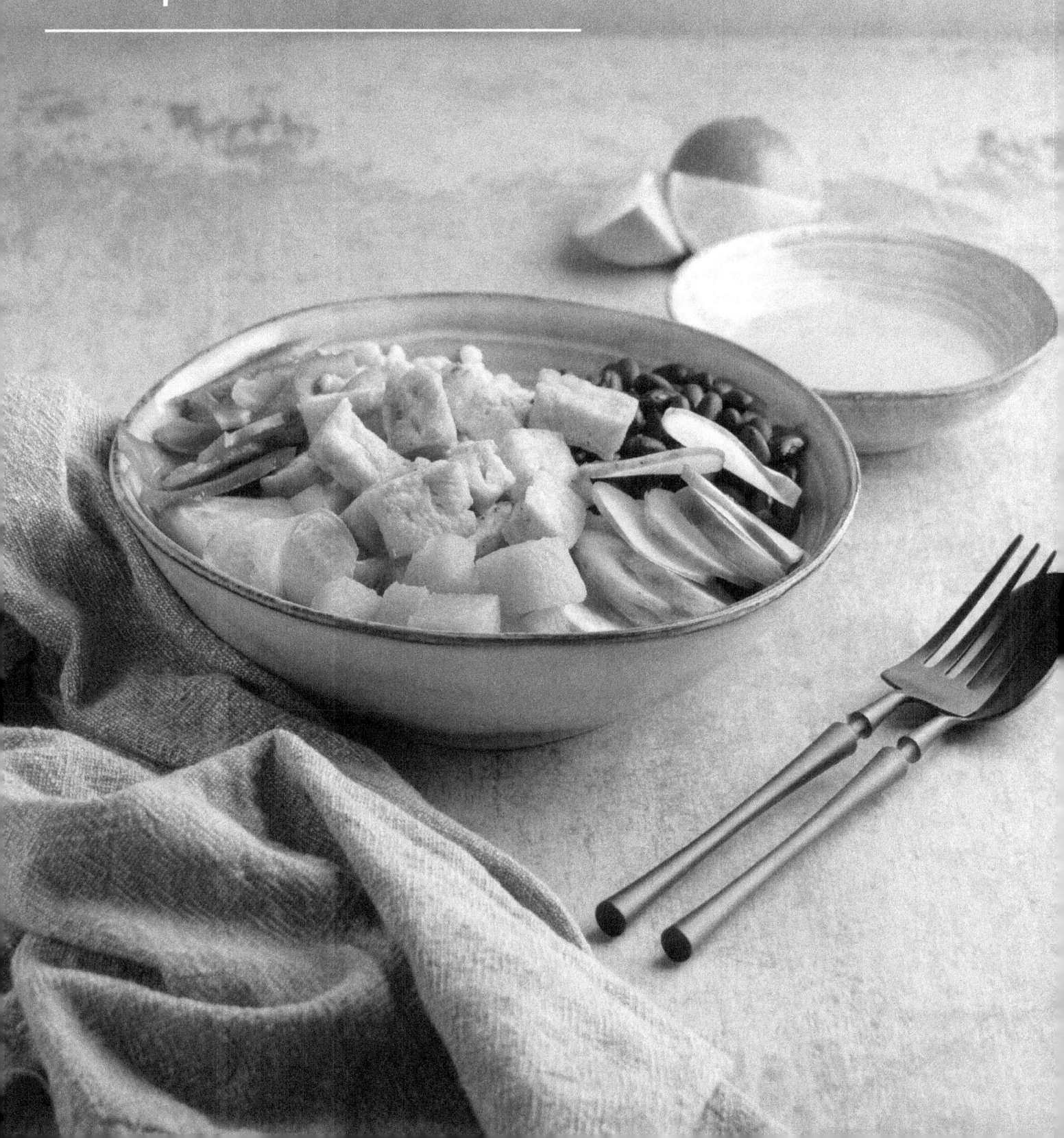

3 6 Zucchini Noodles with Pesto

PREPARATION TIME **15** MIN COOKING TIME **10** MIN SERVINGS **2**

Ingredients

- 2 medium zucchinis, spiralized into noodles
- 1/4 teacup fresh basil leaves
- 1 piece garlic
- 2 tbsps grated Parmesan cheese
- 1 tbsp pine nuts
- 1 tbsp olive oil
- Salt and pepper as needed

Per serving:
Calories: 150kcal;
Fat: 11g;
Carbs: 9g;
Protein: 5g;
Sodium: 85mg;
Potassium: 600mg;
Phosphorus: 75mg

Direction

1. Inside your blending container, blend basil, garlic, Parmesan, pine nuts, and olive oil. Blend 'til you have a smooth pesto sauce.

2. In a pan, sauté the zucchini noodles in a middling temp for around 5mins or 'til they're soft.

3. Shake your zucchini noodles with the pesto sauce and flavour using salt and pepper.

4. Presentinstantly.

3 7 Cauliflower Fried Rice

PREPARATION TIME **15** MIN COOKING TIME **15** MIN SERVINGS **2**

Ingredients

- 2 teacups cauliflower rice (fresh or frozen)
- 1/2 teacupcubed carrots
- 1/2 teacup green peas
- 2 pieces garlic, crushed
- 1 tbsp low-sodium soy sauce
- 1 tsp sesame oil
- 2 eggs, whisked (elective)
- Green onions for garnish (elective)

Per serving:
Calories: 120kcal;
Fat: 4g;
Carbs: 16g;
Protein: 7g;
Sodium: 180mg;
Potassium: 540mg;
Phosphorus: 100mg

Direction

1. Inside your big griddle, sauté the garlic, carrots, and peas in sesame oil till the vegetables are soft.

2. Include cauliflower rice then cook for an extra 5-7 mins.

3. If using eggs, push the cauliflower rice to one side of the griddle and scramble the eggs on the other side.

4. Blend everything in your griddle, include soy sauce, and stir well.

5. Garnish using green onions if anticipated.

3 8 Lemon Garlic Sautéed Asparagus

Ingredients

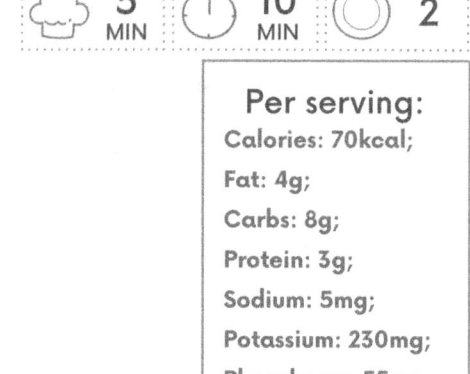

PREPARATION TIME **5** MIN COOKING TIME **10** MIN SERVINGS **2**

- 1 bunch fresh asparagus, clipped
- 1 tbsp olive oil
- 2 pieces garlic, crushed
- Juice of 1 lemon
- Salt and pepper as needed

Per serving:
Calories: 70kcal;
Fat: 4g;
Carbs: 8g;
Protein: 3g;
Sodium: 5mg;
Potassium: 230mg;
Phosphorus: 55mg

Direction

1. Warm olive oil in your pan in a middling temp.
2. Includecrushed garlic and sauté for around 1 min.
3. Include asparagus spears then cook for 5-7 mins or 'til soft-crisp.
4. Squeeze lemon juice over the asparagus, flavour using salt and pepper, then shake to cover.
5. Present hot.

3 9 Roasted Red Peppers Stuffed with Quinoa

Ingredients

PREPARATION TIME **10** MIN COOKING TIME **25** MIN SERVINGS **2**

- 2 big roasted red peppers
- 1/2 teacup cooked quinoa
- 1/4 teacupcubed cucumber
- 1/4 teacupcubed red onion
- 2 tbspssevered fresh parsley
- 1 tbsp lemon juice
- 1 tbsp olive oil
- Salt and pepper as needed

Per serving:
Calories: 200kcal;
Fat: 7g;
Carbs: 29g;
Protein: 5g;
Sodium: 15mg;
Potassium: 270mg;
Phosphorus: 75mg

Direction

1. Inside your container, blend olive oil, salt, cooked quinoa, cucumber, red onion, parsley, lemon juice, and pepper.
2. Stuff the roasted red peppers with the quinoa solution.
3. Put your filled peppers in your baking dish then bake at 350 deg. F for 15-20 mins.
4. Present hot.

4 0 Sautéed Brussels Sprouts with Garlic

Ingredients

PREPARATION TIME 10 MIN · COOKING TIME 10 MIN · SERVINGS 2

- 2 teacups Brussels sprouts, clipped and divided
- 2 pieces garlic, crushed
- 1 tbsp olive oil
- Salt and pepper as needed

Per serving:
Calories: 80kcal;
Fat: 5g;
Carbs: 8g;
Protein: 3g;
Sodium: 30mg;
Potassium: 340mg;
Phosphorus: 60mg

Direction

1. Warm olive oil in your griddle in a med-high temp.
2. Includecrushed garlic and sauté for around 1 min.
3. Include Brussels sprouts then cook for 8-10 mins, or 'til they are soft and mildly browned.
4. Flavour using salt and pepper.
5. Present as a side dish.

4 1 Roasted Butternut Squash Cubes

Ingredients

PREPARATION TIME 10 MIN · COOKING TIME 25 MIN · SERVINGS 2

- 2 teacups butternut squash cubes
- 1 tbsp olive oil
- 1/2 tsp dried thyme
- Salt and pepper as needed

Per serving:
Calories: 90kcal;
Fat: 4g;
Carbs: 16g;
Protein: 1g;
Sodium: 5mg;
Potassium: 450mg;
Phosphorus: 30mg

Direction

1. Warm up your oven to 400deg.F.
2. Shake butternut squash cubes using olive oil, dried thyme, salt, and pepper inside a container.
3. Disperse the seasoned cubes on your baking sheet and roast for 20-25 mins, or 'til they are soft and mildly caramelized.
4. Present hot.

4 2 Cilantro Lime Cauliflower Rice

Ingredients

PREPARATION TIME	COOKING TIME	SERVINGS
10 MIN	10 MIN	2

- 2 teacups cauliflower rice (fresh or frozen)
- 2 tbsps fresh cilantro, severed
- Juice of 1 lime
- 1/4 tsp cumin
- Salt and pepper as needed

Per serving:
Calories: 30kcal;
Fat: 0g;
Carbs: 7g;
Protein: 2g;
Sodium: 30mg;
Potassium: 380mg;
Phosphorus: 40mg

Direction

1. Inside yourgriddle, heat cauliflower rice inside a med-high temp.till it's fully heated.
2. Stir in fresh cilantro, lime juice, cumin, salt, and pepper.
3. Cook for an extra 2-3 mins, mixing irregularly.
4. Present hot.

4 3 Eggplant and Bell Pepper Stir Fry

Ingredients

PREPARATION TIME	COOKING TIME	SERVINGS
10 MIN	15 MIN	2

- 1 small eggplant, cubed
- 1 red bell pepper, carved
- 1 green bell pepper, carved
- 2 pieces garlic, crushed
- 1 tbsp low-sodium soy sauce
- 1 tbsp olive oil
- Salt and pepper as needed

Per serving:
Calories: 90kcal;
Fat: 5g;
Carbs: 12g;
Protein: 2g;
Sodium: 100mg;
Potassium: 380mg;
Phosphorus: 50mg

Direction

1. Warm olive oil in your pan in a med-high temp.
2. Includecrushed garlic and stir-fry for around 30 secs.
3. Includecubed eggplant and carved bell peppers and stir-fry for around 10-12 mins or 'til they are soft.
4. Stir in low-sodium soy sauce and flavour using salt and pepper.
5. Present hot.

4 4 Garlic Butter Mushrooms

PREPARATION TIME 5 MIN   COOKING TIME 10 MIN   SERVINGS 2

Ingredients

- 2 teacups button mushrooms, carved
- 2 pieces garlic, crushed
- 1 tbsp unsalted butter
- 1 tbsp fresh parsley, severed
- Salt and pepper as needed

Per serving:
Calories: 60kcal;
Fat: 4g;
Carbs: 5g;
Protein: 2g;
Sodium: 10mg;
Potassium: 360mg;
Phosphorus: 60mg

Direction

1. Inside yourgriddle, dissolve the unsalted butter in a med-high temp.
2. Includecrushed garlic and sauté for around 1 min.
3. Includecarved mushrooms then cook for 8-10 mins, or 'til they are soft and browned.
4. Flavour using salt and pepper, then garnish with fresh parsley.
5. Present hot.

4 5 Roasted Beets with Orange Glaze

PREPARATION TIME 10 MIN   COOKING TIME 45 MIN   SERVINGS 2

Ingredients

- 2 medium beets, skinned and cubed
- 2 tbsps fresh orange juice
- 1 tsp olive oil
- 1 tsp honey (elective, for sweetness)
- Salt and pepper as needed

Per serving:
Calories: 70kcal;
Fat: 1g;
Carbs: 16g;
Protein: 2g;
Sodium: 80mg;
Potassium: 440mg;
Phosphorus: 40mg

Direction

1. Warm up your oven to 375deg.F.
2. Shake cubed beets using olive oil, fresh orange juice, honey (if using), salt, and pepper inside a container.
3. Disperse the covered beets on your baking sheet and roast for 35-45 mins, or 'til they are soft.
4. Present hot.

4 6 Steamed Artichokes with Olive Oil

PREPARATION TIME 10 MIN   COOKING TIME 30 MIN   SERVINGS 2

Ingredients

- 2 big artichokes
- 1 tbsp olive oil
- Lemon wedges for garnish (elective)
- Salt and pepper as needed

Per serving:
Calories: 90kcal;
Fat: 7g;
Carbs: 7g;
Protein: 2g;
Sodium: 60mg;
Potassium: 370mg;
Phosphorus: 60mg

Direction

1. Trim the tops and stems of your artichokes, and take out any tough outer leaves.
2. Put your artichokes in a steamer basket over boiling water.
3. Cover then steam for approximately 30 mins or 'til the leaves can be simply pulled off.
4. Present using olive oil for soaking, then garnish with lemon wedges if anticipated.
5. Flavour using salt and pepper as needed.

4 7 Lemon Herb Grilled Zucchini

PREPARATION TIME 10 MIN   COOKING TIME 10 MIN   SERVINGS 2

Ingredients

- 2 medium zucchinis, carved lengthwise
- Juice of 1 lemon
- 1 tbsp olive oil
- 1 tsp dried herbs (e.g., thyme or rosemary)
- Salt and pepper as needed

Per serving:
Calories: 70kcal;
Fat: 4g;
Carbs: 8g;
Protein: 2g;
Sodium: 5mg;
Potassium: 420mg;
Phosphorus: 40mg

Direction

1. Warm up grill or your grill pan to med-high temp.
2. Inside your container, blend lemon juice, olive oil, dried herbs, salt, and pepper.
3. Brush the zucchini slices with the lemon herb solution.
4. Grill the zucchini for around 3-4 mins on all sides, or 'til they have grill marks and are soft.
5. Present hot.

4 8 Cabbage and Carrot Slaw

Ingredients

PREPARATION TIME 10 MIN   COOKING TIME 0 MIN   SERVINGS 2

* 2 teacupsteared up cabbage (green or red)
* 1 teacup grated carrots
* 2 tbsps apple cider vinegar
* 1 tbsp olive oil
* 1/2 tsp honey (elective, for sweetness)
* Salt and pepper as needed

Per serving:
Calories: 80kcal;
Fat: 5g;
Carbs: 9g;
Protein: 1g;
Sodium: 30mg;
Potassium: 240mg;
Phosphorus: 20mg

Direction

1. Inside your big container, blendteared up cabbage and grated carrots.
2. Inside your distinct small container, whisk collectively apple cider vinegar, olive oil, honey (if using), salt, and pepper.
3. Pour your dressing over the cabbage and carrot solution then shake to blend.
4. Put in the fridge for almost 30 mins prior to serving.

4 9 Sautéed Green Beans with Almonds

Ingredients

PREPARATION TIME 10 MIN   COOKING TIME 10 MIN   SERVINGS 2

* 2 teacups fresh green beans, clipped
* 2 tbsps slivered almonds
* 1 tbsp olive oil
* 1 piece garlic, crushed
* Salt and pepper as needed

Per serving:
Calories: 100kcal;
Fat: 7g;
Carbs: 8g;
Protein: 2g;
Sodium: 10mg;
Potassium: 220mg;
Phosphorus: 40mg

Direction

1. Warm olive oil in your griddle in a med-high temp.
2. Includecrushed garlic and sauté for around 1 min.
3. Include green beans and slivered almonds, and sauté for 8-10 mins, or 'til the beans are soft-crisp and mildly browned.
4. Flavour using salt and pepper.
5. Present hot.

5 0 Roasted Cauliflower Steaks

PREPARATION TIME	COOKING TIME	SERVINGS
10 MIN	25 MIN	2

Ingredients

- 1 head of cauliflower, carved into thick "steaks"
- 2 tbsps olive oil
- 1 tsp garlic powder
- 1 tsp paprika
- Salt and pepper as needed

Per serving:
Calories: 80kcal;
Fat: 7g;
Carbs: 5g;
Protein: 2g;
Sodium: 30mg;
Potassium: 400mg;
Phosphorus: 50mg

Direction

1. Warm up your oven to 425deg.F.
2. Inside your container, blend olive oil, garlic powder, paprika, salt, and pepper.
3. Brush both sides of your cauliflower steaks using the olive oil solution.
4. Put your cauliflower steaks on your baking sheet and roast for around 20-25 mins, or 'til they are soft and browned.
5. Present hot.

5 1 Sesame Ginger Bok Choy

PREPARATION TIME	COOKING TIME	SERVINGS
10 MIN	10 MIN	2

Ingredients

- 2 baby bok choy heads, divided
- 1 tbsp low-sodium soy sauce
- 1 tsp sesame oil
- 1/2 tsp grated fresh ginger
- 1 piece garlic, crushed
- 1 tsp sesame seeds (elective)
- Salt and pepper as needed

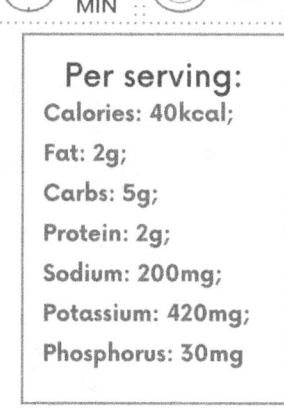

Per serving:
Calories: 40kcal;
Fat: 2g;
Carbs: 5g;
Protein: 2g;
Sodium: 200mg;
Potassium: 420mg;
Phosphorus: 30mg

Direction

1. Warm agriddle in a med-high temp.
2. Include divided bok choy heads, cut side down, then cook for 2-3 mins 'til they start to char.
3. Inside your small container, whisk collectively low-sodium soy sauce, sesame oil, grated ginger, crushed garlic, salt, and pepper.
4. Pour your sauce over the bok choy then cook for an extra 2-3 mins.
5. Garnish using sesame seeds if anticipated and present hot.

5 2 Stuffed Acorn Squash with Wild Rice

PREPARATION TIME | 15 MIN
COOKING TIME | 45 MIN
SERVINGS | 2

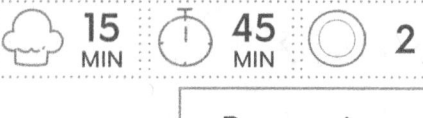

Ingredients

- 1 acorn squash, divided and seeds taken out
- 1/2 teacup cooked wild rice
- 1/4 teacupsevered dried cranberries
- 1/4 teacupsevered pecans
- 1 tbsp olive oil
- 1/2 tsp dried sage
- Salt and pepper as needed

Per serving:
Calories: 280kcal;
Fat: 14g;
Carbs: 41g;
Protein: 5g;
Sodium: 10mg;
Potassium: 810mg;
Phosphorus: 105mg

Direction

1. Warm up your oven to 375deg.F.
2. Brush the inside of the acorn squash halves using olive oil and flavour with dried sage, salt, and pepper.
3. Inside your container, blend cooked wild rice, dried cranberries, and severed pecans.
4. Stuff each acorn squash half with the wild rice solution.
5. Put your filled squash halves on your baking sheet and roast for 35-45 mins or 'til the squash is soft.
6. Present hot.

5 3 Grilled Asparagus with Lemon Zest

PREPARATION TIME | 5 MIN
COOKING TIME | 10 MIN
SERVINGS | 2

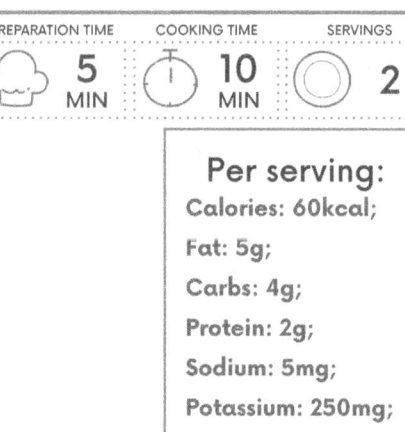

Ingredients

- 1 bunch fresh asparagus, clipped
- 1 tbsp olive oil
- Zest of 1 lemon
- Salt and pepper as needed

Per serving:
Calories: 60kcal;
Fat: 5g;
Carbs: 4g;
Protein: 2g;
Sodium: 5mg;
Potassium: 250mg;
Phosphorus: 40mg

Direction

1. Warm up grill or your grill pan to med-high temp.
2. Shake asparagus spears using olive oil, lemon zest, salt, and pepper.
3. Grill the asparagus for around 5-7 mins, mixing irregularly, 'til they are soft and mildly charred.
4. Present hot.

5 4 Creamy Polenta with Roasted Vegetables

Ingredients

PREPARATION TIME **10** MIN COOKING TIME **30** MIN SERVINGS **2**

- 1/2 teacup cornmeal (polenta)
- 2 teacups water
- 1/4 teacup grated Parmesan cheese
- 1 tbsp olive oil
- 1 teacup roasted mixed vegetables (e.g., bell peppers, zucchini, carrots)
- Salt and pepper as needed

Per serving:
Calories: 240kcal;
Fat: 10g;
Carbs: 32g;
Protein: 7g;
Sodium: 180mg;
Potassium: 320mg;
Phosphorus: 150mg

Direction

1. Inside your saucepot, bring water to a boil. Slowly whisk in your cornmeal.
2. Decrease temp. to low then simmer, mixing regularly, for around 20-25 mins or 'til the polenta thickens.
3. Stir in grated Parmesan cheese, olive oil, salt, and pepper.
4. Present the creamy polenta topped with roasted mixed vegetables.

5 5 Stuffed Bell Peppers with Rice and Veggies

Ingredients

PREPARATION TIME **15** MIN COOKING TIME **40** MIN SERVINGS **2**

- 2 bell peppers, divided and seeds taken out
- 1/2 teacup cooked rice
- 1/4 teacupcubed carrots
- 1/4 teacupcubed zucchini
- 1/4 teacupcubed onions
- 1/4 teacup low-sodium tomato sauce
- 1/2 tsp dried oregano
- Salt and pepper as needed

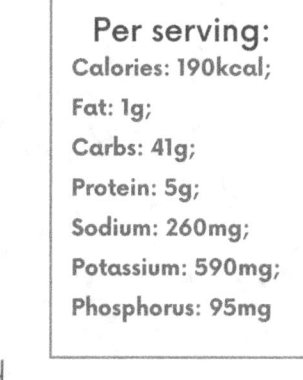

Per serving:
Calories: 190kcal;
Fat: 1g;
Carbs: 41g;
Protein: 5g;
Sodium: 260mg;
Potassium: 590mg;
Phosphorus: 95mg

Direction

1. Warm up your oven to 375deg.F.
2. Inside your container, blend cooked rice, cubed carrots, cubed zucchini, cubed onions, low-sodium tomato sauce, dried oregano, salt, and pepper.
3. Stuff each bell pepper half with the rice and vegetable solution.
4. Put your filled bell peppers in your baking dish and cover with aluminum foil.
5. Bake for a total of 30-35 mins, then take out the foil then bake for an extra 5-10 mins, or 'til the peppers are soft.
6. Present hot.

5 6 Ratatouille with Fresh Basil

Ingredients

PREPARATION TIME **15** MIN　COOKING TIME **30** MIN　SERVINGS **2**

- 1 small eggplant, cubed
- 1 small zucchini, cubed
- 1 small red bell pepper, cubed
- 1 small yellow bell pepper, cubed
- 1 small onion, cubed
- 2 pieces garlic, crushed
- 1 tin (14 oz) low-sodium cubed tomatoes
- 1 tbsp olive oil
- 1/2 tsp dried basil
- Salt and pepper as needed
- Fresh basil leaves for garnish

Per serving:
Calories: 140kcal;
Fat: 6g;
Carbs: 20g;
Protein: 3g;
Sodium: 180mg;
Potassium: 600mg;
Phosphorus: 75mg

Direction

1. Inside your big griddle, warm olive oil inside a middling temp.
2. Includecrushed garlic and cubed onion, and sauté for around 2 mins.
3. Includecubed eggplant, zucchini, red bell pepper, and yellow bell pepper. Sauté for 5-7 mins 'til the vegetables start to soften.
4. Stir in low-sodium cubed tomatoes, dried basil, salt, and pepper. Simmer for 15-20 mins, or 'til the vegetables are soft.
5. Garnish using fresh basil leaves prior to serving.

5 7 Sautéed Snow Peas and Carrots

Ingredients

PREPARATION TIME **10** MIN　COOKING TIME **10** MIN　SERVINGS **2**

- 2 teacups snow peas, clipped
- 1 teacupcarved carrots
- 1 tbsp olive oil
- 1 piece garlic, crushed
- Salt and pepper as needed

Per serving:
Calories: 80kcal;
Fat: 4g;
Carbs: 10g;
Protein: 2g;
Sodium: 25mg;
Potassium: 300mg;
Phosphorus: 45mg

Direction

1. Inside yourgriddle, warm olive oil in a med-high temp.
2. Includecrushed garlic and carved carrots. Sauté for around 3 mins.
3. Include snow peas and continue to sauté for an extra 5-7 mins, or 'til the vegetables are soft-crisp.
4. Flavour using salt and pepper.
5. Present hot.

5 8 Balsamic Glazed Roasted Vegetables

PREPARATION TIME 10 MIN   COOKING TIME 25 MIN   SERVINGS 2

Ingredients

- 2 teacups mixed vegetables (e.g., bell peppers, zucchini, cherry tomatoes)
- 2 tbsps balsamic vinegar
- 1 tbsp olive oil
- 1 piece garlic, crushed
- Salt and pepper as needed

Per serving:
Calories: 90kcal;
Fat: 5g;
Carbs: 10g;
Protein: 2g;
Sodium: 10mg;
Potassium: 350mg;
Phosphorus: 50mg

Direction

1. Warm up your oven to 425deg.F.
2. Inside your container, blend mixed vegetables, balsamic vinegar, olive oil, crushed garlic, salt, and pepper.
3. Disperse the covered vegetables on your baking sheet and roast for 20-25 mins, or 'til they are soft and mildly caramelized.
4. Present hot.

5 9 Quinoa Stuffed Eggplants

Ingredients

PREPARATION TIME 15 MIN   COOKING TIME 35 MIN   SERVINGS 2

- 2 small eggplants
- 1/2 teacup cooked quinoa
- 1/4 teacupcubed tomatoes (tinned, no salt added)
- 1/4 teacupcubed red bell pepper
- 1/4 teacupcubed zucchini
- 1/4 teacupcubed onion
- 1 piece garlic, crushed
- 1/2 tsp dried oregano
- Salt and pepper as needed

Per serving:
Calories: 190kcal;
Fat: 1g;
Carbs: 45g;
Protein: 5g;
Sodium: 25mg;
Potassium: 680mg;
Phosphorus: 115mg

Direction

1. Warm up your oven to 375deg.F.
2. Cut the tops off the eggplants and hollow them out, leaving about a 1/2-inch thick shell.
3. Inside your container, blend cooked quinoa, cubed tomatoes, cubed red bell pepper, cubed zucchini, cubed onion, crushed garlic, dried oregano, salt, and pepper.
4. Stuff each eggplant with the quinoa solution.
5. Put your filled eggplants in your baking dish and cover using aluminum foil. Bake for a total of 30 mins, then take out the foil then bake for an extra 5-10 mins, or 'til the eggplants are soft.
6. Present hot.

6 0 Avocado and Cucumber Sushi Rolls

PREPARATION TIME — **15** MIN   COOKING TIME — **0** MIN   SERVINGS — **2**

Ingredients

- 2 sheets of nori (seaweed)
- 1 teacup cooked and seasoned sushi rice (no added salt)
- 1/2 avocado, carved
- 1/2 cucumber, julienned
- Pickled ginger and low-sodium soy sauce for serving (elective)

Per serving:

Calories: 225kcal;

Fat: 7g;

Carbs: 38g;

Protein: 4g;

Sodium: 15mg;

Potassium: 440mg;

Phosphorus: 85mg

Direction

1. Put your bamboo sushi rolling mat on a clean surface and put a sheet of plastic wrap on top.
2. Lay one sheet of nori on the plastic wrap-covered sushi mat.
3. Wet your fingers using water to prevent the rice from sticking and disperse half of the seasoned sushi rice evenly over your nori, leaving a 1-inch border at the top.
4. Put avocado slices and julienned cucumber in your center of the rice.
5. Carefully roll the nori, using the sushi mat to help you. Seal the roll by moistening the edge with a little water.
6. Repeat the process with the second sheet of nori.
7. Slice each roll into bite-sized pieces and present with pickled ginger and low-sodium soy sauce if anticipated.

* In this recipe limited quantity of avocado is used, compatible with milder forms of CKD. It's essential to consult your doctor about including avocado in your diet! It is possible to replace it with mango or marinated beet.

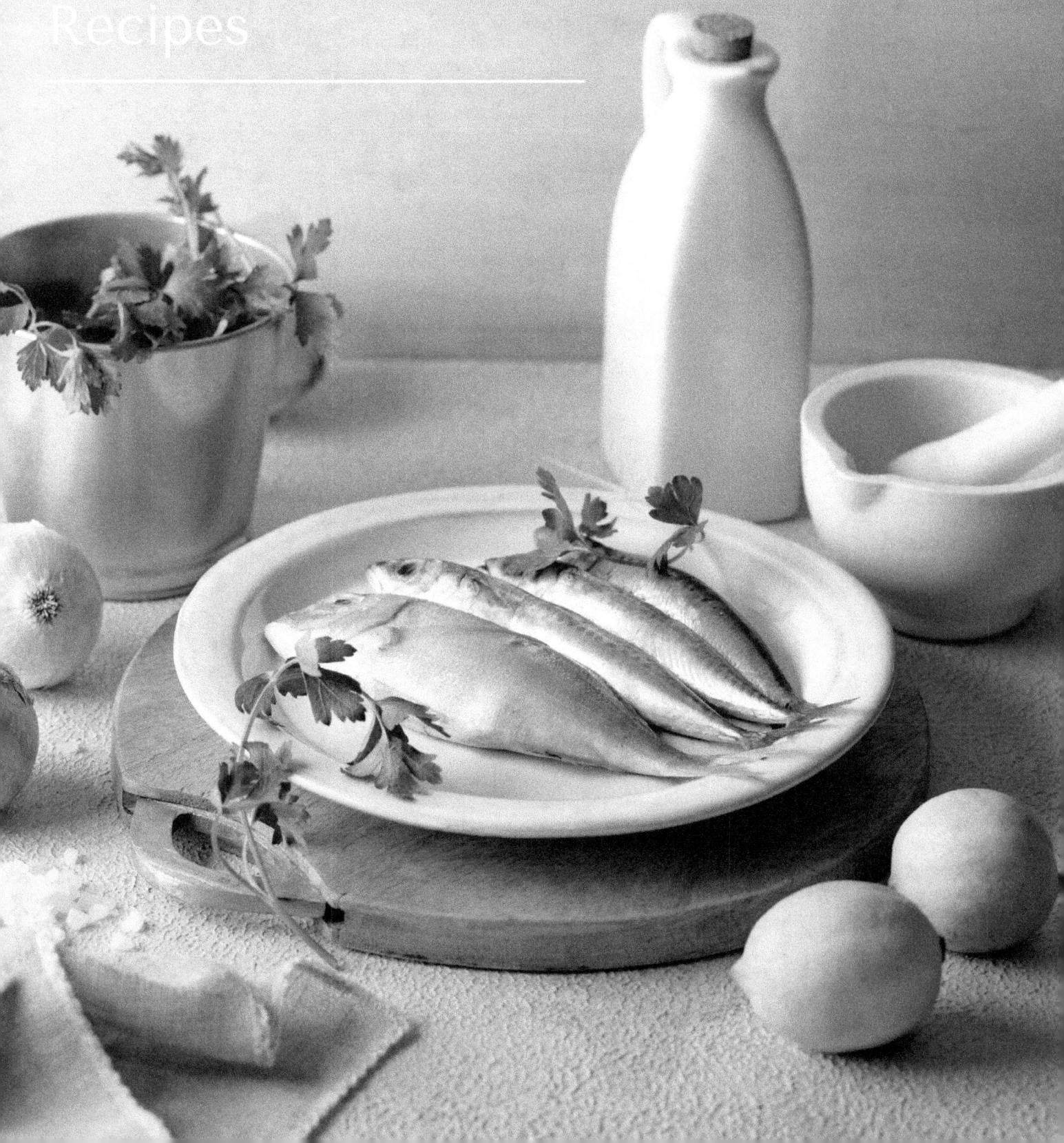

Fish and Seafood

Recipes

6 1 Grilled Salmon with Lemon and Dill

PREPARATION TIME 10 MIN   COOKING TIME 10 MIN   SERVINGS 2

Ingredients

- 2 salmon fillets
- 1 lemon, finelycarved
- 1 tbsp fresh dill, severed
- Olive oil for brushing
- Salt and pepper as needed

Per serving:
Calories: 250kcal;
Fat: 12g;
Carbs: 2g;
Protein: 30g;
Sodium: 150mg;
Potassium: 600mg;
Phosphorus: 250mg

Direction

1. Warm up your grill to med-high temp.
2. Flavour your salmon fillets using salt, pepper, and severed dill.
3. Put lemon slices on top of each fillet.
4. Brush the grill grates using olive oil to prevent sticking.
5. Grill the salmon for around 4-5 mins on all sides or 'til it flakes simply using a fork.
6. Present with a side of your steamed green beans or asparagus.

6 2 Pan-seared Cod with Vegetables

Ingredients

PREPARATION TIME 15 MIN   COOKING TIME 15 MIN   SERVINGS 2

- 2 cod fillets
- 1 zucchini, carved
- 1 red bell pepper, carved
- 1 tbsp olive oil
- 1 tsp dried herbs (e.g., basil, oregano)
- Salt and pepper as needed

Per serving:
Calories: 250kcal;
Fat: 8g;
Carbs: 8g;
Protein: 35g;
Sodium: 150mg;
Potassium: 500mg;
Phosphorus: 250mg

Direction

1. Warm olive oil in your griddle in a med-high temp.
2. Flavour the cod fillets with dried herbs, salt, and pepper.
3. Include cod fillets to the griddle then cook for around 4-5 mins on all sides till they are opaque and flake simply.
4. Inside your another pan, sauté the carved zucchini and red bell pepper till they are soft.
5. Present the pan-seared cod on a bed of sautéed vegetables.

6 3 Baked Tilapia with Garlic and Herb

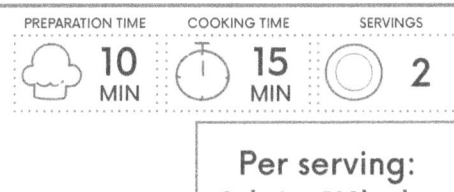

PREPARATION TIME 10 MIN COOKING TIME 15 MIN SERVINGS 2

Ingredients

- 2 tilapia fillets
- 2 pieces garlic, crushed
- 1 tbsp fresh parsley, severed
- 1 tbsp lemon juice
- Salt and pepper as needed

Per serving:
Calories: 180kcal;
Fat: 3g;
Carbs: 2g;
Protein: 35g;
Sodium: 120mg;
Potassium: 400mg;
Phosphorus: 200mg

Direction

1. Warm up your oven to 375deg.F.
2. Put tilapia fillets in your baking dish.
3. Spraycrushed garlic, severed parsley, and lemon juice over the fillets.
4. Flavour using salt and pepper.
5. Cover the baking dish using foil then bake for 15 mins or 'til the fish flakes simply using a fork.
6. Present with a side of steamed broccoli.

6 4 Lemon Butter Shrimp

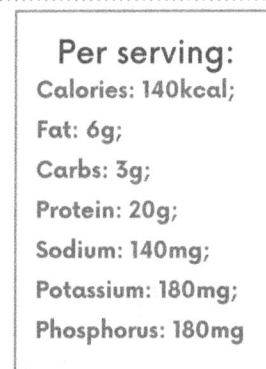

PREPARATION TIME 10 MIN COOKING TIME 10 MIN SERVINGS 2

Ingredients

- 12 big shrimp, skinned and deveined
- 1 tbsp unsalted butter
- 1 lemon, juiced and zested
- 1 piece garlic, crushed
- 1 tbsp fresh parsley, severed
- Salt and pepper as needed

Per serving:
Calories: 140kcal;
Fat: 6g;
Carbs: 3g;
Protein: 20g;
Sodium: 140mg;
Potassium: 180mg;
Phosphorus: 180mg

Direction

1. Warm butter in your griddle in a middling temp.
2. Includecrushed garlic then cook for around 1 mintill fragrant.
3. Include shrimp then cook for 2-3 mins on all sides till they turn pink.
4. Stir in lemon juice and zest, severed parsley, salt, and pepper.
5. Present hot with a side salad.

65 Grilled Tuna Steaks with Salsa

PREPARATION TIME | 15 MIN
COOKING TIME | 8 MIN
SERVINGS | 2

Ingredients

- 2 tuna steaks
- 1/2 teacupcubed cucumber
- 1/2 teacupcubed red onion
- 1/2 teacupcubed bell pepper
- 1 tbsp fresh cilantro, severed
- 1 tbsp lime juice
- Salt and pepper as needed

Per serving:
Calories: 220kcal;
Fat: 4g;
Carbs: 8g;
Protein: 38g;
Sodium: 180mg;
Potassium: 600mg;
Phosphorus: 350mg

Direction

1. Warm up your grill to med-high temp.
2. Flavour the tuna steaks using salt and pepper.
3. Grill the tuna steaks for around 3-4 mins on all sides for medium-rare doneness.
4. Inside your container, blendcubed cucumber, red onion, bell pepper, cilantro, and lime juice to make the salsa.
5. Present the grilled tuna steaks topped with the fresh salsa.

66 Broiled Sole with Lemon Parsley Sauce

PREPARATION TIME | 10 MIN
COOKING TIME | 10 MIN
SERVINGS | 2

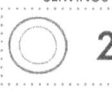

Ingredients

- 2 sole fillets
- 1 lemon, juiced and zested
- 2 tbsps fresh parsley, severed
- 1 tbsp olive oil
- Salt and pepper as needed

Per serving:
Calories: 180kcal;
Fat: 7g;
Carbs: 3g;
Protein: 26g;
Sodium: 150mg;
Potassium: 300mg;
Phosphorus: 180mg

Direction

1. Warm up your broiler.
2. Put sole fillets on a broiler pan.
3. Inside your small container, blend lemon juice, lemon zest, severed parsley, olive oil, salt, and pepper.
4. Brush the lemon parsley sauce over the sole fillets.
5. Broil for around 4-5 mins or 'til the fish flakes simply.
6. Present with a side of your steamed green beans.

6 7 Sautéed Scallops with Garlic

Ingredients

PREPARATION TIME 10 MIN   **COOKING TIME** 5 MIN   **SERVINGS** 2

- 12 scallops
- 2 pieces garlic, crushed
- 1 tbsp olive oil
- 1 tbsp fresh parsley, severed
- Salt and pepper as needed

Per serving:
Calories: 150kcal;
Fat: 5g;
Carbs: 3g;
Protein: 23g;
Sodium: 180mg;
Potassium: 340mg;
Phosphorus: 210mg

Direction

1. Warm olive oil in your griddle in a med-high temp.
2. Includecrushed garlic then cook for around 1 mintill fragrant.
3. Flavour scallops using salt and pepper.
4. Include scallops to the griddle and sauté for around 2-3 mins on all sides till they are mildly browned.
5. Spray with severed parsley prior to serving.
6. Present with a side of sautéed spinach.

6 8 Baked Haddock with Roasted Vegetables

Ingredients

PREPARATION TIME 15 MIN   **COOKING TIME** 20 MIN   **SERVINGS** 2

- 2 haddock fillets
- 1 zucchini, carved
- 1 red bell pepper, carved
- 1 onion, carved
- 1 tbsp olive oil
- 1 tsp dried thyme
- Salt and pepper as needed

Per serving:
Calories: 220kcal;
Fat: 7g;
Carbs: 10g;
Protein: 30g;
Sodium: 180mg;
Potassium: 600mg;
Phosphorus: 250mg

Direction

1. Warm up your oven to 375deg.F.
2. Put haddock fillets in your baking dish.
3. Inside your container, shake carved zucchini, red bell pepper, and onion using olive oil, dried thyme, salt, and pepper.
4. Organize the vegetable solution around the haddock fillets in your baking dish.
5. Bake for around 20 mins or 'til the fish flakes simply and the vegetables are soft.
6. Present hot.

6 9 Lemon Herb Grilled Trout

Ingredients

PREPARATION TIME   COOKING TIME   SERVINGS

10 MIN   **10** MIN   **2**

- 2 trout fillets
- 1 lemon, juiced and zested
- 2 tbsps fresh herbs (e.g., parsley, thyme, rosemary), severed
- 1 tbsp olive oil
- Salt and pepper as needed

Per serving:
Calories: 250kcal;
Fat: 12g;
Carbs: 3g;
Protein: 30g;
Sodium: 170mg;
Potassium: 500mg;
Phosphorus: 200mg

Direction

1. Warm up your grill to med-high temp.
2. Inside your small container, blend lemon juice, lemon zest, severed herbs, olive oil, salt, and pepper.
3. Brush the lemon herb solution over the trout fillets.
4. Grill the trout for around 4-5 mins on all sides or 'til it flakes simply.
5. Present with a side of steamed asparagus.

7 0 Steamed Clams with Garlic Broth

Ingredients

PREPARATION TIME   COOKING TIME   SERVINGS
10 MIN   **10** MIN   **2**

- 24 littleneck clams, scrubbed
- 2 pieces garlic, crushed
- 1 teacup low-sodium chicken broth
- 2 tbsps fresh parsley, severed
- Salt and pepper as needed

Per serving:
Calories: 180kcal;
Fat: 2g;
Carbs: 6g;
Protein: 30g;
Sodium: 170mg;
Potassium: 300mg;
Phosphorus: 180mg

Direction

1. Inside your big pot, heat chicken broth in a med-high temp.
2. Includecrushed garlic and raise the broth to a simmer.
3. Include clams to the pot and cover with a lid.
4. Steam for around 5-7 mins or 'til the clams open.
5. Discard any unopened clams.
6. Spray with severed parsley and flavour using salt and pepper.
7. Present the clams with a side of steamed broccoli.

7 1 Poached Salmon with Asparagus

PREPARATION TIME 10 MIN · COOKING TIME 15 MIN · SERVINGS 2

Ingredients

- 2 salmon fillets
- 1 bunch of asparagus, clipped
- 1 lemon, finelycarved
- 2 teacups low-sodium chicken broth
- Fresh dill for garnish
- Salt and pepper as needed

Per serving:
Calories: 250kcal;
Fat: 10g;
Carbs: 8g;
Protein: 30g;
Sodium: 250mg;
Potassium: 600mg;
Phosphorus: 250mg

Direction

1. Inside your big griddle, raise the chicken broth to a simmer.
2. Flavour the salmon fillets using salt and pepper.
3. Put your salmon fillets and lemon slices in your simmering broth.
4. Include asparagus to the griddle, ensuring they are partially submerged.
5. Cover and poach for around 10-12 mins or 'til the salmon flakes simply.
6. Garnish using fresh dill and present hot.

7 2 Shrimp Stir Fry with Mixed Vegetables

PREPARATION TIME 15 MIN · COOKING TIME 10 MIN · SERVINGS 2

Ingredients

- 12 big shrimp, skinned and deveined
- 2 teacups mixed vegetables (e.g., broccoli, bell peppers, snap peas)
- 1 piece garlic, crushed
- 1 tbsp low-sodium soy sauce
- 1 tbsp olive oil
- Salt and pepper as needed

Per serving:
Calories: 180kcal;
Fat: 7g;
Carbs: 12g;
Protein: 20g;
Sodium: 220mg;
Potassium: 400mg;
Phosphorus: 200mg

Direction

1. Warm olive oil in your griddle in a med-high temp.
2. Includecrushed garlic and sauté for around 1 mintill fragrant.
3. Include shrimp and stir-fry for 2-3 mins 'til pink.
4. Include mixed vegetables and stir-fry for an extra 4-5 mins 'til soft.
5. Stir in low-sodium soy sauce, salt, and pepper.
6. Present hot.

7 3 Cod Cakes with Garlic Aioli

PREPARATION TIME	COOKING TIME	SERVINGS
15 MIN	15 MIN	2

Ingredients

For Cod Cakes:
- 2 cod fillets
- 1/2 teacup breadcrumbs (use whole grain breadcrumbs if preferred)
- 1 egg
- 1/4 teacup finely severed onion
- 1 tbsp fresh parsley, severed
- Salt and pepper as needed

For Garlic Aioli:
- 2 pieces garlic, crushed
- 1/4 teacup Greek yogurt (low-fat)
- 1 tsp lemon juice
- Salt and pepper as needed

Per serving:
Calories: 300kcal;
Fat: 8g;
Carbs: 25g;
Protein: 30g;
Sodium: 260mg;
Potassium: 500mg;
Phosphorus: 250mg

Direction

For Cod Cakes:
1. Cook the cod fillets by baking or grilling till they are flaky.
2. Flake the cooked cod into a bowl.
3. Include breadcrumbs, egg, severed onion, parsley, salt, and pepper.
4. Blend thoroughly and form into patties.
5. Warm your non-stick griddle in a med-high temp.
6. Cook the cod cakes for around 3-4 mins on all sides till golden brown.

For Garlic Aioli:
7. Inside your small container, blend crushed garlic, Greek yogurt, lemon juice, salt, and pepper.
8. Mix till well blended.
9. Present the cod cakes with a side of garlic aioli.

7 4 Herb-Crusted Tilapia with Lemon

PREPARATION TIME	COOKING TIME	SERVINGS
10 MIN	12 MIN	2

Ingredients

- 2 tilapia fillets
- 1/2 teacup whole wheat breadcrumbs
- 1 tbsp fresh parsley, severed
- 1 tsp dried thyme
- 1 tsp dried rosemary
- 1 lemon, juiced
- 1 tbsp olive oil
- Salt and pepper as needed

Per serving:
Calories: 220kcal;
Fat: 8g;
Carbs: 14g;
Protein: 25g;
Sodium: 260mg;
Potassium: 350mg;
Phosphorus: 180mg

Direction

1. Warm up your oven to 375deg.F.
2. In a shallow dish, blend breadcrumbs, severed parsley, dried thyme, dried rosemary, salt, and pepper.
3. Brush the tilapia fillets with lemon juice and olive oil.
4. Coat each fillet with the breadcrumb solution, pressing it on to adhere.
5. Put your covered fillets on your baking sheet.
6. Bake for around 10-12 mins or 'til the fish flakes simply.
7. Present with lemon wedges.

7 5 Grilled Mackerel with Orange Glaze

Ingredients

PREPARATION TIME — 10 MIN   COOKING TIME — 10 MIN   SERVINGS — 2

- 2 mackerel fillets
- 1 orange, juiced and zested
- 2 tbsps low-sodium soy sauce
- 1 tbsp honey
- 1 tsp grated ginger
- Salt and pepper as needed

Per serving:
Calories: 280kcal;
Fat: 15g;
Carbs: 14g;
Protein: 24g;
Sodium: 220mg;
Potassium: 400mg;
Phosphorus: 250mg

Direction

1. Inside your container, blend orange juice, orange zest, low-sodium soy sauce, honey, grated ginger, salt, and pepper to make the glaze.
2. Warm up your grill to med-high temp.
3. Brush the mackerel fillets with the glaze.
4. Grill the mackerel for around 4-5 mins on all sides or 'til it flakes simply.
5. Brush with additional glaze while grilling if anticipated

In this recipe limited quantity of avocado is used, compatible with milder forms of CKD. It's essential to consult your doctor about including avocado in your diet! It is possible to replace it with mango or marinated beet.

7 6 Baked Catfish with Cajun Spice

Ingredients

PREPARATION TIME — 10 MIN   COOKING TIME — 20 MIN   SERVINGS — 2

- 2 catfish fillets
- 1 tbsp Cajun spice mix (low-sodium)
- 1 lemon, juiced
- 1 tbsp olive oil
- Salt and pepper as needed

Per serving:
Calories: 250kcal;
Fat: 11g;
Carbs: 3g;
Protein: 31g;
Sodium: 180mg;
Potassium: 400mg;
Phosphorus: 250mg

Direction

1. Warm up your oven to 375deg.F.
2. Flavour catfish fillets with Cajun spice mix, salt, and pepper.
3. Spray with lemon juice and olive oil.
4. Put your catfish on your baking sheet.
5. Bake for around 15-20 mins or 'til the fish flakes simply.
6. Present with a side of steamed broccoli or green beans.

7 7 Seared Tuna with Avocado Salad

Ingredients

PREPARATION TIME 15 MIN   COOKING TIME 5 MIN   SERVINGS 2

- 2 tuna steaks
- 1 avocado, cubed
- 1 cucumber, cubed
- 1 tomato, cubed
- 1/4 red onion, finely severed
- 1 tbsp fresh cilantro, severed
- 1 lime, juiced
- Salt and pepper as needed

Per serving:
Calories: 280kcal;
Fat: 14g;
Carbs: 14g;
Protein: 28g;
Sodium: 180mg;
Potassium: 800mg;
Phosphorus: 250mg

Direction

1. Flavour tuna steaks using salt and pepper.
2. Warm yournon-stick griddle in a med-high temp.
3. Sear tuna steaks for around 2-3 mins on all sides till they are seared on the outside but still pink in your center.
4. Inside your container, blend lime juice, salt, cubed avocado, cucumber, tomato, red onion, cilantro, and pepper to make the salad.
5. Present the seared tuna steaks with avocado salad.

7 8 Lemon Garlic Roasted Shrimp

Ingredients

PREPARATION TIME 10 MIN   COOKING TIME 10 MIN   SERVINGS 2

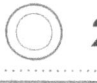

- 12 big shrimp, skinned and deveined
- 2 pieces garlic, crushed
- 1 lemon, juiced and zested
- 1 tbsp olive oil
- Fresh parsley for garnish
- Salt and pepper as needed

Per serving:
Calories: 180kcal;
Fat: 8g;
Carbs: 4g;
Protein: 24g;
Sodium: 180mg;
Potassium: 220mg;
Phosphorus: 180mg

Direction

1. Warm up your oven to 400deg.F.
2. Inside your container, blendcrushed garlic, lemon juice, lemon zest, olive oil, salt, and pepper.
3. Shake shrimp in your solution to cover evenly.
4. Disperse the shrimp on your baking sheet.
5. Roast for around 8-10 mins 'til the shrimp turn pink and opaque.
6. Garnish using fresh parsley prior to serving.

7 9 Steamed Lobster with Drawn Butter

Ingredients

	PREPARATION TIME	COOKING TIME	SERVINGS

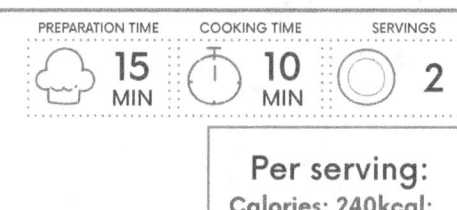

- 2 lobster tails
- 4 tbsps unsalted butter
- 1 lemon, juiced
- Salt and pepper as needed

Per serving:
Calories: 280kcal;
Fat: 22g;
Carbs: 2g;
Protein: 18g;
Sodium: 350mg;
Potassium: 350mg;
Phosphorus: 180mg

Direction

1. Fill your big pot with around an inch of water and raise it to a boil.
2. Put a steamer basket over the pot.
3. Cut the lobster tails in half lengthwise.
4. Steam the lobster tails for around 12-15 mins 'til the meat turns white and opaque.
5. Inside your small saucepan, dissolve unsalted butter at low heat.
6. Stir in your lemon juice, salt, and pepper to make the drawn butter.
7. Present the steamed lobster with drawn butter for soaking.

8 0 Pan-seared Halibut with Mango Salsa

Ingredients

- 2 halibut fillets
- 1 ripe mango, cubed
- 1/4 red onion, finely severed
- 1/4 red bell pepper, cubed
- 1 tbsp fresh cilantro, severed
- 1 lime, juiced
- Salt and pepper as needed

Per serving:
Calories: 240kcal;
Fat: 2g;
Carbs: 25g;
Protein: 30g;
Sodium: 170mg;
Potassium: 680mg;
Phosphorus: 250mg

Direction

1. Flavour halibut fillets using salt and pepper.
2. Warm yournon-stick griddle in a med-high temp.
3. Pan-sear halibut fillets for around 3-4 mins on all sides till they are thoroughly cooked and mildly browned.
4. Inside your container, blendcubed mango, red onion, red bell pepper, cilantro, lime juice, salt, and pepper to make the salsa.
5. Present the pan-seared halibut with mango salsa.

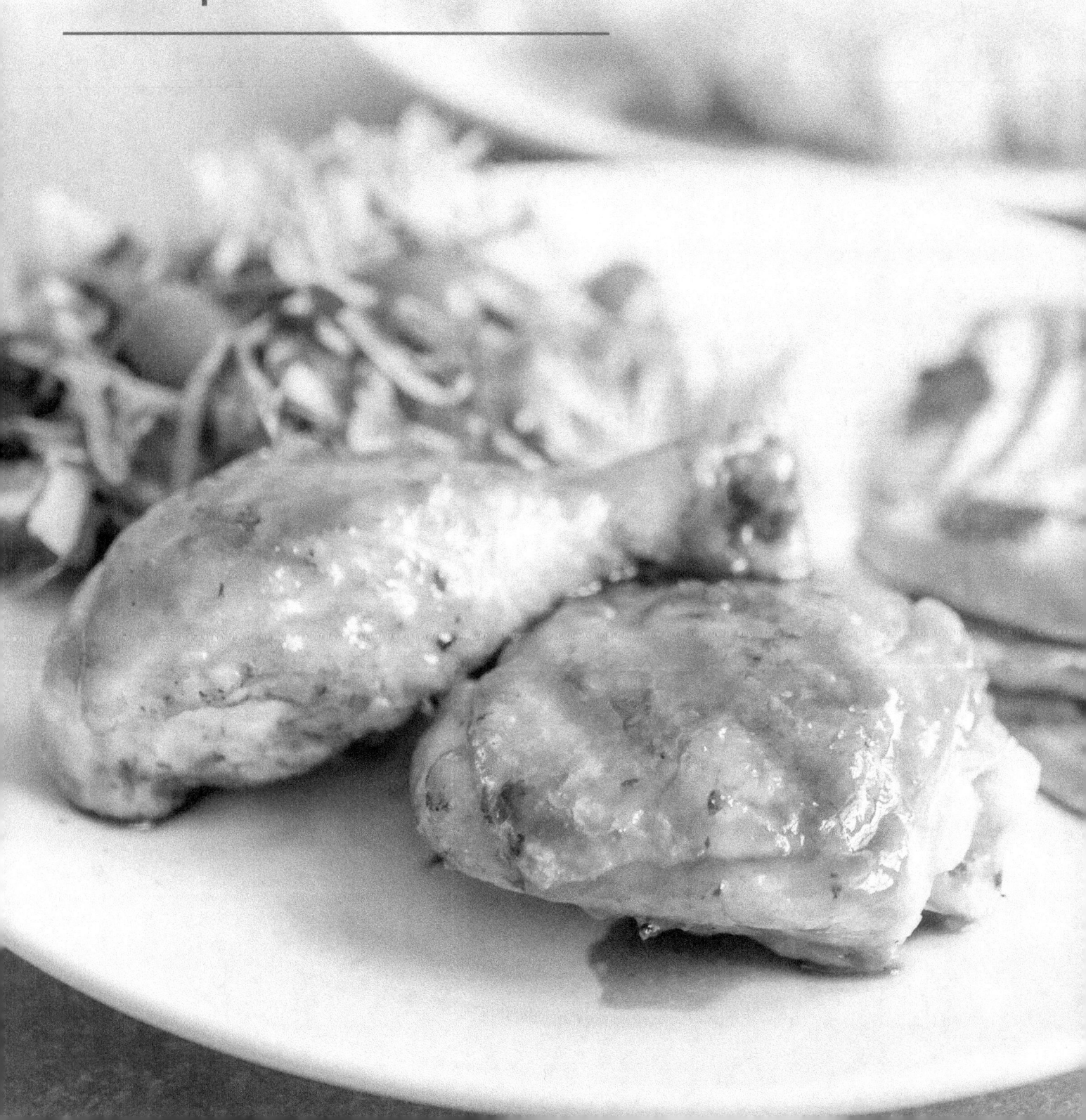

Meat
Recipes

8 1 Lemon Herb Grilled Chicken

PREPARATION TIME **10** MIN   COOKING TIME **15** MIN   SERVINGS **2**

Ingredients

- 2 boneless, skinless chicken breasts
- 1 lemon, juiced and zested
- 1 tsp olive oil
- 1 tsp dried oregano
- 1 tsp dried thyme
- Salt and pepper as needed

Per serving:
Calories: 180kcal;
Fat: 5g;
Carbs: 3g;
Protein: 30g;
Sodium: 150mg;
Potassium: 380mg;
Phosphorus: 260mg

Direction

1. Inside your small container, blend lemon juice, lemon zest, olive oil, dried oregano, dried thyme, salt, and pepper to make a marinade.
2. Put chicken breasts in your zip-top bag and pour the marinade over them. Seal the bag then put in the fridge for almost 30 mins.
3. Warm up a grill to med-high temp.
4. Grill the chicken for around 6-7 mins on all sides, or 'til the internal temp. reaches 165deg.F.
5. Present the grilled chicken with your favorite renal-friendly vegetables.

8 2 Baked Turkey Breast with Herbs

Ingredients

PREPARATION TIME **10** MIN   COOKING TIME **30** MIN   SERVINGS **2**

- 2 turkey breast fillets
- 1 tsp olive oil
- 1 tsp dried rosemary
- 1 tsp dried thyme
- Salt and pepper as needed

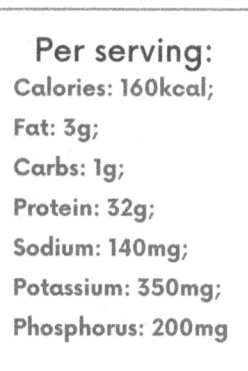

Per serving:
Calories: 160kcal;
Fat: 3g;
Carbs: 1g;
Protein: 32g;
Sodium: 140mg;
Potassium: 350mg;
Phosphorus: 200mg

Direction

1. Warm up your oven to 375deg.F.
2. Brush turkey breast fillets using olive oil and flavour with dried rosemary, dried thyme, salt, and pepper.
3. Put your seasoned turkey fillets on your baking sheet.
4. Bake for around 25-30 mins, or 'til the internal temp. reaches 165deg.F.
5. Let it rest for a couple of mins prior to serving with renal-friendly sides.

8 3 Pork Tenderloin with Apples

Ingredients

PREPARATION TIME   10 MIN   COOKING TIME   25 MIN   SERVINGS   2

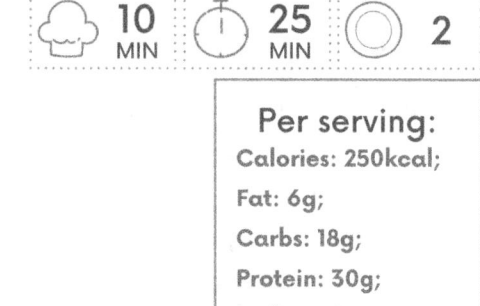

- 1 pork softloin (about 1 lb.)
- 2 apples, skinned, cored, and carved
- 1 tsp olive oil
- 1 tsp dried sage
- Salt and pepper as needed

Per serving:
Calories: 250kcal;
Fat: 6g;
Carbs: 18g;
Protein: 30g;
Sodium: 200mg;
Potassium: 450mg;
Phosphorus: 230mg

Direction

1. Warm up your oven to 375deg.F.
2. Flavour the pork softloin with dried sage, salt, and pepper.
3. Warm olive oil in an oven-safe griddle in a med-high temp. Sear the pork softloin on all sides 'til browned.
4. Includecarved apples to the griddle.
5. Transfer the griddle to the warmed up oven then bake for around 20-25 mins or 'til your pork reaches an internal temp. of 145 deg. F.
6. Slice the pork and present with the cooked apples.

This recipe uses pork, compatible with milder forms of CKD. It's essential to consult your doctor about including pork in your diet.

8 4 Grilled Lamb Chops with Rosemary

Ingredients

PREPARATION TIME   10 MIN   COOKING TIME   10 MIN   SERVINGS   2

- 4 lamb chops
- 1 tsp olive oil
- 1 tsp dried rosemary
- Salt and pepper as needed

Per serving:
Calories: 320kcal;
Fat: 23g;
Carbs: 0g;
Protein: 28g;
Sodium: 120mg;
Potassium: 340mg;
Phosphorus: 200mg

Direction

1. Warm up a grill to med-high temp.
2. Brush lamb chops using olive oil and flavour with dried rosemary, salt, and pepper.
3. Grill the lamb chops for around 4-5 mins on all sides for medium-rare, adjusting the time for your preferred doneness.
4. Let them rest for a couple ofmins prior to serving with renal-friendly vegetables.

8 5 Beef Stir Fry with Broccoli

Ingredients

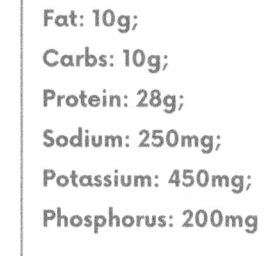

PREPARATION TIME **15** MIN COOKING TIME **15** MIN SERVINGS **2**

- 8 oz lean beef strips
- 2 teacups broccoli florets
- 1 tsp low-sodium soy sauce
- 1 tsp crushed ginger
- 1 tsp crushed garlic
- 1 tsp olive oil

Per serving:
Calories: 250kcal;
Fat: 10g;
Carbs: 10g;
Protein: 28g;
Sodium: 250mg;
Potassium: 450mg;
Phosphorus: 200mg

Direction

1. In a wok or griddle, warm olive oil at high temp.
2. Includecrushed ginger and garlic, sauté for around 30 secs.
3. Include beef strips and stir-fry 'til browned.
4. Include broccoli florets and continue to stir-fry for an extra 3-4 mins 'til the broccoli is soft-crisp.
5. Stir in low-sodium soy sauce then cook for an extra min.
6. Present hot with a side of renal-friendly rice or noodles

This recipe uses red meat, compatible with milder forms of CKD. It's essential to consult your doctor about including red meat in your diet

8 6 Chicken Kabobs with Vegetables

Ingredients

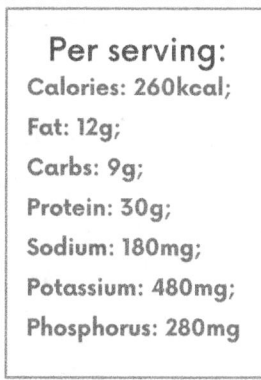

PREPARATION TIME **15** MIN COOKING TIME **15** MIN SERVINGS **2**

- 2 boneless, skinless chicken breasts, that is cut into chunks
- 1 bell pepper, that is cut into chunks
- 1 zucchini, carved
- 1 red onion, that is cut into chunks
- 2 tbsp olive oil
- 1 tsp dried basil
- 1 tsp dried oregano
- Salt and pepper as needed

Per serving:
Calories: 260kcal;
Fat: 12g;
Carbs: 9g;
Protein: 30g;
Sodium: 180mg;
Potassium: 480mg;
Phosphorus: 280mg

Direction

1. Inside your container, mix olive oil, dried basil, dried oregano, salt, and pepper.
2. Thread the chicken, bell pepper, zucchini, and red onion onto skewers.
3. Brush the skewers using the olive oil solution.
4. Grill your kabobs on med-high temp.for around 6-8 mins on all sides or 'til the chicken is thoroughly cooked.
5. Present with your favorite renal-friendly side dish.

8 7 Balsamic Glazed Chicken Breast

Ingredients

PREPARATION TIME **10** MIN   COOKING TIME **20** MIN   SERVINGS **2**

- 2 boneless, skinless chicken breasts
- 2 tbsp balsamic vinegar
- 1 tbsp olive oil
- 1 tsp dried rosemary
- 1 tsp honey (elective, for sweetness)
- Salt and pepper as needed

Per serving:
Calories: 230kcal;
Fat: 9g;
Carbs: 3g;
Protein: 32g;
Sodium: 180mg;
Potassium: 360mg;
Phosphorus: 210mg

Direction

1. Inside your container, blend balsamic vinegar, olive oil, dried rosemary, honey (if anticipated), salt, and pepper.
2. Coat the chicken breasts with the balsamic solution.
3. Warm agriddle in a med-high temp. then cook the chicken for around 8-10 mins on all sides or 'til done.
4. Present with a renal-friendly vegetable or salad.

8 8 Pork Chops with Sautéed Apples

Ingredients

PREPARATION TIME **10** MIN   COOKING TIME **20** MIN   SERVINGS **2**

- 2 pork chops
- 2 apples, skinned, cored, and carved
- 1 tsp olive oil
- 1 tsp dried sage
- Salt and pepper as needed

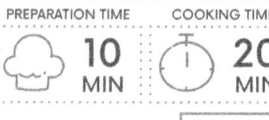

Per serving:
Calories: 280kcal;
Fat: 10g;
Carbs: 16g;
Protein: 30g;
Sodium: 140mg;
Potassium: 360mg;
Phosphorus: 230mg

Direction

1. Flavour the pork chops with dried sage, salt, and pepper.
2. Warm olive oil in your griddle in a med-high temp. Sear the pork chops on both sides 'til browned.
3. Include the carved apples to the griddle then cook for around 5-7 mins 'til they are soft.
4. Present the pork chops with sautéed apples and a renal-friendly side dish.

This recipe uses pork, compatible with milder forms of CKD. It's essential to consult your doctor about including pork in your diet.

8 9 Roast Beef with Steamed Vegetables

Ingredients

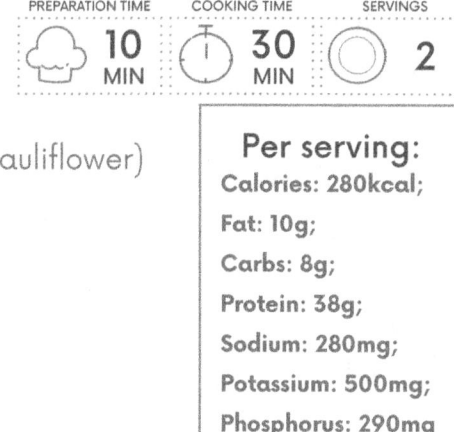

PREPARATION TIME 10 MIN
COOKING TIME 30 MIN
SERVINGS 2

- 8 oz roast beef slices
- 2 teacups mixed steamed vegetables (e.g., broccoli, carrots, cauliflower)
- 1 tsp olive oil
- 1 tsp dried thyme
- Salt and pepper as needed

Per serving:
Calories: 280kcal;
Fat: 10g;
Carbs: 8g;
Protein: 38g;
Sodium: 280mg;
Potassium: 500mg;
Phosphorus: 290mg

Direction

1. Warm up your oven to 350deg.F.
2. Put your roast beef slices in your baking dish.
3. Spray olive oil over the beef and flavour with dried thyme, salt, and pepper.
4. Bake for around 20-25 mins 'til fully heated.
5. Present with steamed vegetables on the side.

This recipe uses red meat, compatible with milder forms of CKD. It's essential to consult your doctor about including beef in your diet!

9 0 Garlic Butter Baked Chicken Thighs

Ingredients

PREPARATION TIME 10 MIN
COOKING TIME 35 MIN
SERVINGS 2

- 4 bone-in, skinless chicken thighs
- 2 tbsp unsalted butter, dissolved
- 2 pieces garlic, crushed
- 1 tsp dried thyme
- Salt and pepper as needed

Per serving:
Calories: 330kcal;
Fat: 23g;
Carbs: 1g;
Protein: 29g;
Sodium: 140mg;
Potassium: 320mg;
Phosphorus: 210mg

Direction

1. Warm up your oven to 375deg.F.
2. Mix dissolved butter, crushed garlic, dried thyme, salt, and pepper inside a container.
3. Coat the chicken thighs with the garlic butter solution.
4. Put your chicken thighs in your baking dish then bake for around 30-35 mins 'til the chicken is thoroughly cooked.
5. Present with renal-friendly vegetables or a side salad.

9 1 Grilled Veal with Lemon and Capers

Ingredients

PREPARATION TIME **15** MIN　COOKING TIME **10** MIN　SERVINGS **2**

- 2 veal cutlets
- 1 lemon, juiced and zested
- 2 tsp capers
- 1 tsp olive oil
- 1 tsp dried thyme
- Salt and pepper as needed

Per serving:
Calories: 240kcal;
Fat: 8g;
Carbs: 3g;
Protein: 38g;
Sodium: 180mg;
Potassium: 320mg;
Phosphorus: 280mg

Direction

1. Inside your small container, blend lemon juice, lemon zest, capers, olive oil, dried thyme, salt, and pepper to make a marinade.
2. Brush the veal cutlets with the marinade.
3. Warm up a grill to med-high temp.
4. Grill the veal for around 4-5 mins on all sides or 'til cooked to your desired doneness.
5. Present the grilled veal with a side of renal-friendly vegetables.

9 2 Sautéed Duck Breast with Orange Sauce

Ingredients

 PREPARATION TIME **10** MIN COOKING TIME **20** MIN SERVINGS  **2**

- 2 duck breast fillets
- 1 orange, juiced and zested
- 1 tsp olive oil
- 1 tsp honey (elective, for sweetness)
- Salt and pepper as needed

Per serving:
Calories: 300kcal;
Fat: 12g;
Carbs: 6g;
Protein: 38g;
Sodium: 140mg;
Potassium: 400mg;
Phosphorus: 280mg

Direction

1. Score the skin of your duck breasts in a crisscross pattern. Flavour using salt and pepper.
2. Warm olive oil in your griddle in a med-high temp.Put your duck breasts skin-side down then cook for around 6-7 mins 'til the skin is crispy.
3. Flip the duck breasts then cook for an extra 4-5 mins or 'til they reach your desired doneness.
4. Take out the duck breasts from the griddle then let them rest.
5. In the same griddle, include orange juice, orange zest, honey (if anticipated), and any remaining juices from resting the duck. Simmer for a couple ofmins to create the sauce.
6. Slice the duck and spray the orange sauce over it prior to serving.

In this recipe limited quantity of orange is used, compatible with milder forms of CKD. It's essential to consult your doctor about including orange in your diet. It is possible to replace orange with lemon or cranberries.

93 Oven Roasted Cornish Hen

Ingredients

PREPARATION TIME	COOKING TIME	SERVINGS
10 MIN	50 MIN	2

- 2 Cornish hens
- 1 tsp olive oil
- 1 tsp dried rosemary
- Salt and pepper as needed

Per serving:
Calories: 320kcal;
Fat: 18g;
Carbs: 0g;
Protein: 40g;
Sodium: 160mg;
Potassium: 380mg;
Phosphorus: 290mg

Direction

1. Warm up your oven to 375deg.F.
2. Rub the Cornish hens using olive oil and flavour with dried rosemary, salt, and pepper.
3. Put your hens in a roasting pan and roast for around 45-50 mins or 'til they reach an internal temp. of 165deg.F.
4. Let the hens rest for a couple ofmins prior to serving with renal-friendly sides.

94 Pork Loin Roast with Veggies

Ingredients

PREPARATION TIME	COOKING TIME	SERVINGS
15 MIN	45 MIN	2

- 1 pork loin roast (about 1 lb.)
- 2 teacups mixed vegetables (e.g., carrots, green beans, bell peppers)
- 1 tsp olive oil
- 1 tsp dried thyme
- Salt and pepper as needed

Per serving:
Calories: 320kcal;
Fat: 12g;
Carbs: 10g;
Protein: 40g;
Sodium: 190mg;
Potassium: 500mg;
Phosphorus: 310mg

Direction

1. Warm up your oven to 375deg.F.
2. Put your pork loin roast in a roasting pan.
3. Spray olive oil over the roast and flavour with dried thyme, salt, and pepper.
4. Organize the mixed vegetables around the roast.
5. Roast for around 40-45 mins or 'til the pork reaches an internal temp. of 145 deg. F and the vegetables are soft.
6. Slice the pork then present with the roasted vegetables.

*** This recipe uses pork, compatible with milder forms of CKD. It's essential to consult your doctor about including pork in your diet.**

9 5 Skillet Chicken with Lemon and Olives

PREPARATION TIME
 10 MIN

COOKING TIME
 20 MIN

SERVINGS
2

Ingredients

- 2 boneless, skinless chicken thighs
- 1 lemon, juiced and zested
- 1/4 teacupcarved green olives
- 1 tsp olive oil
- 1 tsp dried thyme
- Salt and pepper as needed

Per serving:
Calories: 280kcal;
Fat: 12g;
Carbs: 6g;
Protein: 32g;
Sodium: 190mg;
Potassium: 320mg;
Phosphorus: 230mg

Direction

1. Flavour the chicken thighs with dried thyme, salt, and pepper.
2. Warm olive oil in your griddle in a med-high temp. Cook the chicken thighs for around 6-8 mins on all sides or 'til thoroughly cooked.
3. Take out the chicken from your griddle then put away.
4. In the same griddle, include lemon juice, lemon zest, and carved green olives. Cook for a couple ofmins to create a sauce.
5. Return the chicken to the griddle and cover with the lemon and olive sauce.
6. Present hot with renal-friendly side dishes.

Salad and Dressing
Recipes

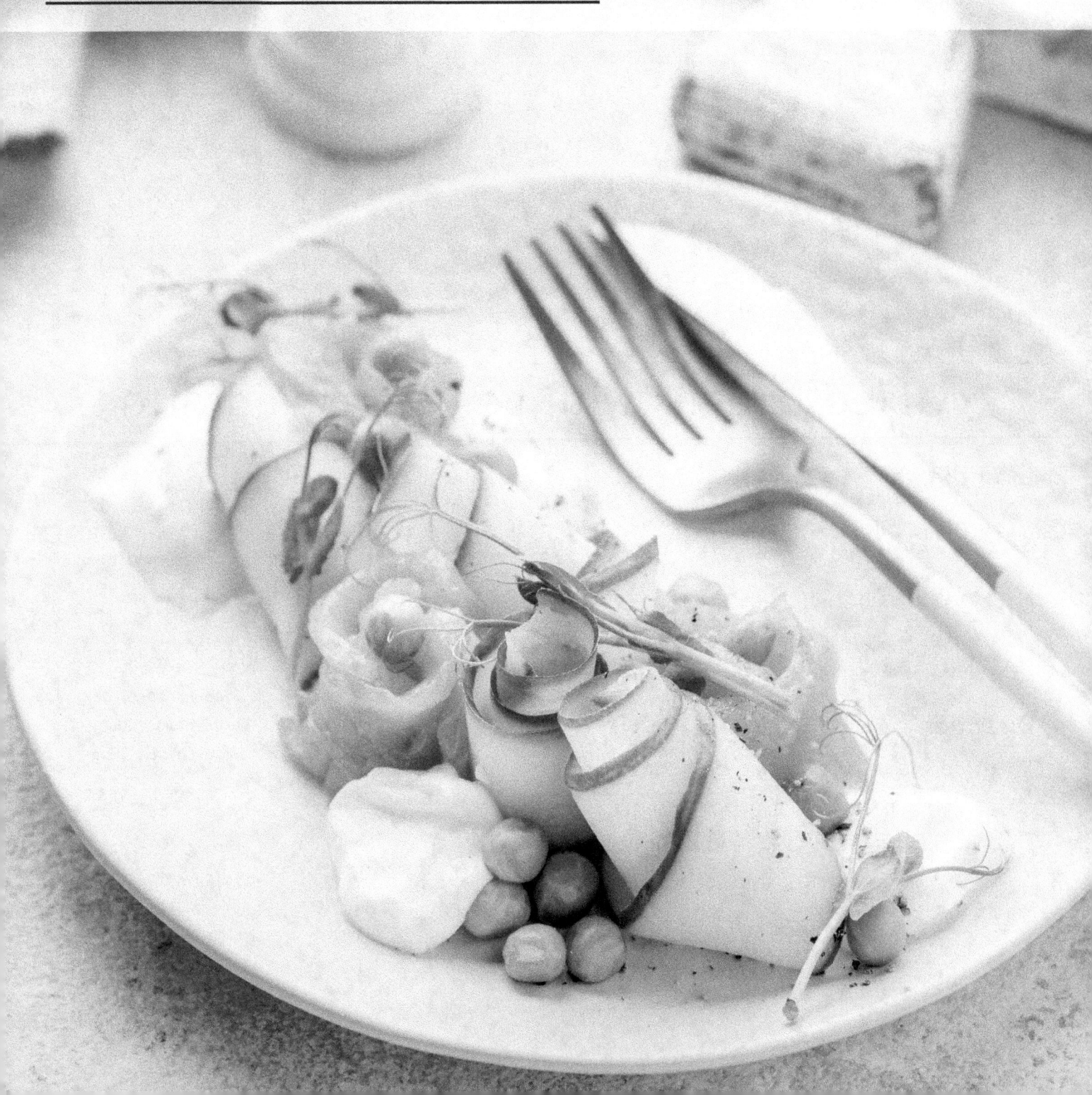

9 6 Cucumber and Dill Salad

Ingredients

PREPARATION TIME   COOKING TIME   SERVINGS

10 MIN   0 MIN   2

- 2 cucumbers, finelycarved
- 2 tbsps fresh dill, severed
- 1/4 teacup red onion, finelycarved
- 2 tbsps olive oil
- 2 tbsps white wine vinegar
- Salt and pepper as needed

Per serving:
Calories: 110kcal;
Fat: 9g;
Carbs: 6g;
Protein: 1g;
Sodium: 10mg;
Potassium: 250mg;
Phosphorus: 20mg

Direction

1. Inside your container, blend the carved cucumbers, severed dill, and carved red onion.
2. Inside your small container, whisk collectively the olive oil and white wine vinegar.
3. Pour your dressing over the cucumber solution then shake to blend.
4. Flavour using salt and pepper as needed.
5. Present chilled

9 7 Mixed Greens with Lemon Vinaigrette

Ingredients

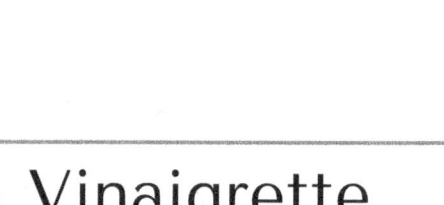

PREPARATION TIME   COOKING TIME   SERVINGS

10 MIN   0 MIN   2

- 4 teacups mixed greens (e.g., lettuce, arugula, and spinach)
- 2 tbsps lemon juice
- 2 tbsps olive oil
- 1/2 tsp honey (elective for sweetness)
- Salt and pepper as needed

Per serving:
Calories: 80kcal;
Fat: 7g;
Carbs: 4g;
Protein: 1g;
Sodium: 20mg;
Potassium: 100mg;
Phosphorus: 20mg

Direction

1. Inside your big container, blend the mixed greens.
2. Inside your small container, whisk collectively the lemon juice, olive oil, honey (if using), salt, and pepper.
3. Spray your dressing over the mixed greens then shake to cover.
4. Presentinstantly

9 8 Kale and Apple Salad

PREPARATION TIME 15 MIN   COOKING TIME 0 MIN   SERVINGS 2

Ingredients

- 2 teacups baby kale (or regular kale with stems taken out), severed
- 1 apple, finelycarved
- 2 tbsps lemon juice
- 1 tbsp olive oil
- 1 tbsp honey (elective)
- Salt and pepper as needed

Per serving:
Calories: 120kcal;
Fat: 4g;
Carbs: 22g;
Protein: 2g;
Sodium: 25mg;
Potassium: 380mg;
Phosphorus: 45mg

Direction

1. Inside your big container, blend the severed kale and carved apple.
2. Inside your small container, whisk collectively the lemon juice, olive oil, honey (if using), salt, and pepper.
3. Spray your dressing over the salad then shake to cover.
4. Allow it to relax for a couple ofmins to soften the kale mildly prior to serving.

9 9 Shaved Fennel and Orange Salad

PREPARATION TIME 10 MIN   COOKING TIME 0 MIN   SERVINGS 2

Ingredients

- 1 fennel bulb, finelycarved
- 1 orange, skinned and segmented
- 2 tbsps fresh orange juice
- 1 tbsp olive oil
- Salt and pepper as needed

Per serving:
Calories: 80kcal;
Fat: 4g;
Carbs: 12g;
Protein: 1g;
Sodium: 25mg;
Potassium: 360mg;
Phosphorus: 30mg

Direction

1. Inside your container, blend the shaved fennel and orange segments.
2. Inside your small container, whisk collectively the fresh orange juice, olive oil, salt, and pepper.
3. Spray your dressing over the salad then shake to blend.
4. Present chilled.

100 Arugula and Pear Salad

Ingredients

- 4 teacups arugula
- 1 ripe pear, finelycarved
- 2 tbsps balsamic vinegar
- 2 tbsps olive oil
- Salt and pepper as needed

PREPARATION TIME	COOKING TIME	SERVINGS
10 MIN	0 MIN	2

Per serving:
Calories: 140kcal;
Fat: 11g;
Carbs: 12g;
Protein: 1g;
Sodium: 20mg;
Potassium: 220mg;
Phosphorus: 20mg

Direction

1. Inside your big container, blend the arugula and carved pear.
2. Inside your small container, whisk collectively the balsamic vinegar, olive oil, salt, and pepper.
3. Spray your dressing over the salad then shake to cover.
4. Presentinstantly.

101 Roasted Beet and Walnut Salad

Ingredients

- 2 medium beets, roasted, skinned, and cubed
- 1/4 teacup walnuts, severed
- 2 teacups mixed greens
- 1 tbsp olive oil
- 1 tbsp balsamic vinegar
- Salt and pepper as needed

PREPARATION TIME	COOKING TIME	SERVINGS
15 MIN	45 MIN	2

Per serving:
Calories: 180kcal;
Fat: 13g;
Carbs: 14g;
Protein: 3g;
Sodium: 70mg;
Potassium: 360mg;
Phosphorus: 70mg

Direction

1. Warm up your oven to 400deg.F. Wrap your beets in aluminum foil then roast for around 45 mins or 'til soft. Let them cool, peel, and dice.
2. Inside your big container, blend the cubed roasted beets, severed walnuts, and mixed greens.
3. Inside your small container, whisk collectively the olive oil and balsamic vinegar.
4. Spray your dressing over the salad then shake to cover.
5. Flavour using salt and pepper as needed.
6. Present at room temp.

102 Cabbage and Carrot Coleslaw

Ingredients

PREPARATION TIME 15 MIN   COOKING TIME 0 MIN   SERVINGS 2

- 2 teacupsteared up cabbage
- 1 teacupteared up carrots
- 2 tbsps plain Greek yogurt
- 1 tbsp apple cider vinegar
- 1 tsp honey (elective for sweetness)
- Salt and pepper as needed

Per serving:
Calories: 70kcal;
Fat: 0g;
Carbs: 16g;
Protein: 2g;
Sodium: 40mg;
Potassium: 280mg;
Phosphorus: 35mg

Direction

1. Inside your big container, blend the teared up cabbage and carrots.
2. Inside your small container, whisk collectively the Greek yogurt, apple cider vinegar, honey (if using), salt, and pepper.
3. Pour your dressing over the coleslaw then shake to cover.
4. Present chilled.

103 Grilled Veggie Salad with Balsamic Glaze

Ingredients

PREPARATION TIME 15 MIN   COOKING TIME 10 MIN   SERVINGS 2

- 2 teacups mixed grilled vegetables (e.g., zucchini, bell peppers, and eggplant)
- 1 tbsp olive oil
- 2 tbsps balsamic glaze
- Salt and pepper as needed

Per serving:
Calories: 100kcal;
Fat: 5g;
Carbs: 13g;
Protein: 2g;
Sodium: 20mg;
Potassium: 350mg;
Phosphorus: 45mg

Direction

1. Warm up grill or your grill pan in a med-high temp. Grill the mixed vegetables tillsoft and mildly charred, around 10mins.
2. Inside your big container, shake the grilled vegetables using olive oil and balsamic glaze.
3. Flavour using salt and pepper as needed.
4. Present warm or at room temp.

104 Mixed Berry Salad with Mint

PREPARATION TIME **10** MIN COOKING TIME **0** MIN SERVINGS **2**

Ingredients

- 1 teacup mixed berries (e.g., strawberries, blueberries, and raspberries)
- 2 tbsps fresh mint leaves, severed
- 1 tsp honey (elective for sweetness)

Per serving:
Calories: 40kcal;
Fat: 0g;
Carbs: 10g;
Protein: 1g;
Sodium: 0mg;
Potassium: 100mg;
Phosphorus: 10mg

Direction

1. Inside your container, blend the mixed berries and severed mint leaves.
2. Spray honey (if using) over the berries and carefully shake to cover.
3. Present chilled.

105 Romaine and Radish Salad

PREPARATION TIME **10** MIN COOKING TIME **0** MIN SERVINGS **2**

Ingredients

- 2 teacups romaine lettuce, severed
- 1 teacupcarved radishes
- 1 tbsp olive oil
- 1 tbsp lemon juice
- Salt and pepper as needed

Per serving:
Calories: 70kcal;
Fat. 7g;
Carbs: 2g;
Protein: 1g;
Sodium: 20mg;
Potassium: 170mg;
Phosphorus: 20mg

Direction

1. Inside your big container, blend the severed romaine lettuce and carved radishes.
2. Inside your small container, whisk collectively the olive oil and lemon juice.
3. Spray your dressing over the salad then shake to cover.
4. Flavour using salt and pepper as needed.
5. Presentinstantly.

106 Sliced Pear and Walnut Salad

Ingredients

PREPARATION TIME · 10 MIN   COOKING TIME · 0 MIN   SERVINGS · 2

- 2 ripe pears, finelycarved
- 1/4 teacup walnuts, severed
- 2 teacups mixed greens
- 2 tbsps olive oil
- 1 tbsp white wine vinegar
- Salt and pepper as needed

Per serving:
Calories: 250kcal;
Fat: 17g;
Carbs: 23g;
Protein: 2g;
Sodium: 10mg;
Potassium: 210mg;
Phosphorus: 40mg

Direction

1. Inside your big container, blend the carved pears, severed walnuts, and mixed greens.
2. Inside your small container, whisk collectively the olive oil and white wine vinegar.
3. Spray your dressing over the salad then shake to cover.
4. Flavour using salt and pepper as needed.
5. Presentinstantly.

107 Watermelon and Feta Salad

Ingredients

PREPARATION TIME · 10 MIN   COOKING TIME · 0 MIN   SERVINGS · 2

- 2 teacups cubed watermelon
- 1/4 teacup crumbled feta cheese
- 2 tbsps fresh mint leaves, severed
- 1 tbsp balsamic vinegar
- Salt and pepper as needed

Per serving:
Calories: 90kcal;
Fat: 3g;
Carbs: 15g;
Protein: 2g;
Sodium: 120mg;
Potassium: 200mg;
Phosphorus: 40mg

Direction

1. Inside your container, blend the cubed watermelon, crumbled feta cheese, and severed fresh mint.
2. Spray balsamic vinegar over the salad then shake carefully to blend.
3. Flavour using salt and pepper as needed.
4. Present chilled.

108 Cilantro Lime Quinoa Salad

PREPARATION TIME 15 MIN   COOKING TIME 15 MIN   SERVINGS 2

Ingredients

- 1 teacup cooked quinoa, cooled
- 1/4 teacup fresh cilantro, severed
- 2 tbsps lime juice
- 1 tbsp olive oil
- Salt and pepper as needed

Per serving:
Calories: 210kcal;
Fat: 7g;
Carbs: 31g;
Protein: 5g;
Sodium: 5mg;
Potassium: 150mg;
Phosphorus: 100mg

Direction

1. Inside your container, blend the cooked and cooled quinoa with severed cilantro.
2. Inside your small container, whisk collectively the lime juice and olive oil.
3. Spray your dressing over the quinoa salad then shake to cover.
4. Flavour using salt and pepper as needed.
5. Present at room temp. or chilled.

109 Summer Squash and Zucchini Salad

PREPARATION TIME 15 MIN   COOKING TIME 0 MIN   SERVINGS 2

Ingredients

- 2 teacupsfinelycarved summer squash and zucchini
- 1/4 teacup fresh basil leaves, torn
- 2 tbsps lemon juice
- 1 tbsp olive oil
- Salt and pepper as needed

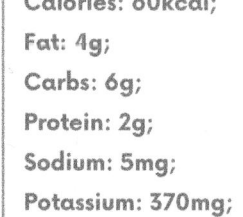

Per serving:
Calories: 60kcal;
Fat: 4g;
Carbs: 6g;
Protein: 2g;
Sodium: 5mg;
Potassium: 370mg;
Phosphorus: 45mg

Direction

1. Inside your container, blend the carved summer squash, zucchini, and torn basil leaves.
2. Inside your small container, whisk collectively the lemon juice and olive oil.
3. Spray your dressing over the salad then shake to blend.
4. Flavour using salt and pepper as needed.
5. Presentinstantly.

110   Greek Salad with Lemon Oregano Dressing

PREPARATION TIME	COOKING TIME	SERVINGS
15 MIN	0 MIN	2

Ingredients

- 2 teacups mixed greens
- 1/2 cucumber, finelycarved
- 1/4 red onion, finelycarved
- 1/4 teacup crumbled feta cheese
- 2 tbsps lemon juice
- 1 tbsp olive oil
- 1/2 tsp dried oregano
- Salt and pepper as needed

Per serving:
Calories: 150kcal;
Fat: 11g;
Carbs: 9g;
Protein: 5g;
Sodium: 170mg;
Potassium: 240mg;
Phosphorus: 85mg

Direction

1. Inside your big container, blend the mixed greens, carved cucumber, red onion, and crumbled feta cheese.

2. Inside your small container, whisk collectively the dried oregano, salt, lemon juice, olive oil, and pepper.

3. Spray your dressing over the salad then shake to cover.

4. Presentinstantly

111   Honey Mustard Chicken Salad

PREPARATION TIME	COOKING TIME	SERVINGS
20 MIN	15 MIN	2

Ingredients

- For the Salad:
- 2 boneless, skinless chicken breasts
- 4 teacups mixed greens
- 1/4 teacup red onion, finelycarved
- 1/4 teacupcarved almonds

- For the Honey Mustard Dressing:
- 2 tbsps Dijon mustard
- 1 tbsp honey
- 1 tbsp olive oil
- 1 tbsp apple cider vinegar
- Salt and pepper as needed

Per serving:
Calories: 350kcal;
Fat: 14g;
Carbs: 24g;
Protein: 32g;
Sodium: 210mg;
Potassium: 580mg;
Phosphorus: 290mg

Direction

1. Flavour the chicken breasts using salt and pepper. Grill or cook them in your griddletillthoroughly cooked, about 6-8 mins on all sides. Let them rest for a couple ofmins prior to slicing.
2. Inside your big container, blend the mixed greens, carved red onion, and carved almonds.
3. Inside your distinct container, whisk collectively the apple cider vinegar, salt, Dijon mustard, honey, olive oil, and pepper to make the dressing.
4. Spray your dressing over the salad then shake to cover.
5. Top the salad with carved chicken.
6. Presentinstantly.

112   Asian Cabbage Slaw with Sesame Dressing

PREPARATION TIME 15 MIN   COOKING TIME 0 MIN   SERVINGS 2

Ingredients

- For the Slaw:
- 4 teacupsfinelycarved cabbage (Napa or regular)
- 1 teacupteared up carrots
- 2 green onions, finelycarved
- 1/4 teacupsevered fresh cilantro
- For the Sesame Dressing:
- 2 tbsps rice vinegar
- 1 tbsp sesame oil
- 1 tbsp low-sodium soy sauce
- 1 tsp honey (elective)
- 1/2 tsp grated fresh ginger
- 1/4 tsp crushed red pepper flakes

Per serving:
Calories: 150kcal;
Fat: 9g;
Carbs: 15g;
Protein: 3g;
Sodium: 240mg;
Potassium: 400mg;
Phosphorus: 65mg

Direction

1. Inside your big container, blend the carved green onions, carved cabbage, teared up carrots, and severed cilantro.
2. Inside your distinct container, whisk collectively the rice vinegar, sesame oil, low-sodium soy sauce, honey (if using), grated ginger, and crushed red pepper flakes (if using).
3. Spray the sesame dressing over the slaw then shake to cover.
4. Presentinstantly

113   Caesar Salad with Grilled Chicken

PREPARATION TIME 20 MIN   COOKING TIME 15 MIN   SERVINGS 2

Ingredients

- For the Salad:
- 2 boneless, skinless chicken breasts
- 4 teacups romaine lettuce, severed
- 1/4 teacup croutons (made without whole grains)
- 1/4 teacupcarved cucumber
- 1/4 teacupcarved red bell pepper
- For the Non-Dairy Caesar Dressing:
- 2 tbsps olive oil
- 1 tbsp lemon juice
- 1 piece garlic, crushed
- 1/2 tsp Dijon mustard
- Salt and pepper as needed

Per serving:
Calories: 320kcal;
Fat: 17g;
Carbs: 12g;
Protein: 29g;
Sodium: 360mg;
Potassium: 620mg;
Phosphorus: 280mg

Direction

1. Flavour the chicken breasts using salt and pepper. Grill or cook them in your griddletillthoroughly cooked, about 6-8 mins on all sides. Let them rest for a couple ofmins prior to slicing.
2. Inside your big container, blend the severed romaine lettuce, croutons, carved cucumber, and carved red bell pepper.
3. Inside your distinct container, whisk collectively the olive oil, lemon juice, crushed garlic, Dijon mustard, salt, and pepper to make the non-dairy Caesar dressing.
4. Spray your dressing over the salad then shake to cover.
5. Top the salad with carved chicken.
6. Presentinstantly.

114 Raspberry Vinaigrette Mixed Green Salad

PREPARATION TIME	COOKING TIME	SERVINGS
10 MIN	0 MIN	2

Ingredients

- For the Salad:
- 4 teacups mixed greens
- 1/4 teacupcarved red onion
- 1/4 teacupsevered pecans
- 1/2 teacup fresh raspberries

- For the Raspberry Vinaigrette:
- 2 tbsps raspberry vinegar
- 2 tbsps olive oil
- 1 tsp honey (elective)
- Salt and pepper as needed

Per serving:
Calories: 220kcal;
Fat: 17g;
Carbs: 15g;
Protein: 3g;
Sodium: 20mg;
Potassium: 280mg;
Phosphorus: 45mg

Direction

1. Inside your big container, blend the mixed greens, carved red onion, severed pecans, and fresh raspberries.
2. Inside your distinct container, whisk collectively the raspberry vinegar, olive oil, honey (if using), salt, and pepper to make the raspberry vinaigrette.
3. Spray your dressing over the salad then shake to cover.
4. Presentinstantly.

115 Roasted Cauliflower and Arugula Salad

PREPARATION TIME	COOKING TIME	SERVINGS
15 MIN	20 MIN	2

Ingredients

- For the Salad:
- 4 teacups arugula
- 2 teacups roasted cauliflower florets
- 1/4 teacupcarved red onion
- 1/4 teacupsevered fresh parsley
- For the Lemon Vinaigrette:

- 2 tbsps lemon juice
- 2 tbsps olive oil
- 1 tsp Dijon mustard
- Salt and pepper as needed

Per serving:
Calories: 160kcal;
Fat: 12g;
Carbs: 12g;
Protein: 4g;
Sodium: 120mg;
Potassium: 600mg;
Phosphorus: 70mg

Direction

1. Warm up your oven to 425deg.F. Shake your cauliflower florets with a little olive oil, salt, and pepper. Roast for around 20 mins or 'til soft and mildly golden. Let them cool.
2. Inside your big container, blend the arugula, roasted cauliflower florets, carved red onion, and severed fresh parsley.
3. Inside your distinct container, whisk collectively the Dijon mustard, salt, lemon juice, olive oil, and pepper to make the lemon vinaigrette.
4. Spray your dressing over the salad then shake to cover.
5. Present at room temp.

Dessert
Recipes

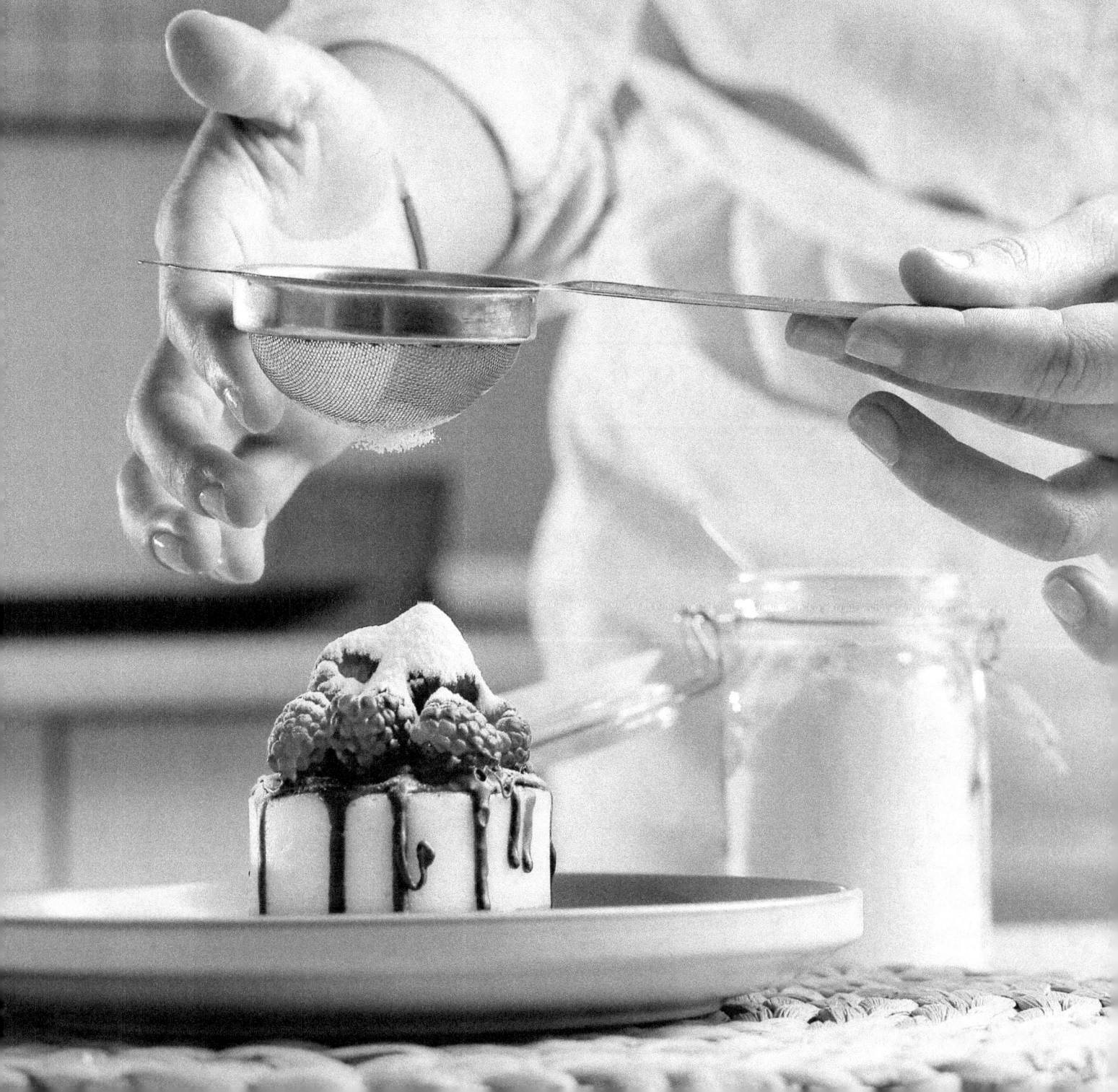

116 Berry Sorbet

Ingredients

PREPARATION TIME 5 MIN   COOKING TIME 0 MIN   SERVINGS 2

- 1 teacup mixed berries (strawberries, blueberries, raspberries)
- 1/2 teacup unsweetened applesauce
- 1/2 tsp lemon juice
- Stevia or erythritol (elective, for added sweetness)

Per serving:
Calories: 50kcal;
Fat: 0g;
Carbs: 13g;
Protein: 0g;
Sodium: 0mg;
Potassium: 100mg;
Phosphorus: 10mg

Direction

1. Inside a mixer, blend the mixed berries, unsweetened applesauce, and lemon juice.
2. Blend 'til smooth.
3. Taste then include a small amount of stevia or erythritol if anticipated for sweetness.
4. Pour your solution into a container and freeze for almost 2 hrs.
5. Present as a refreshing sorbet

117 Baked Apples with Cinnamon

Ingredients

PREPARATION TIME 10 MIN   COOKING TIME 30 MIN   SERVINGS 2

- 2 apples (choose low-potassium varieties like Granny Smith)
- 1/2 tsp ground cinnamon
- 1 tsp honey (elective, use sparingly)

Per serving:
Calories: 80kcal;
Fat: 0g;
Carbs: 22g;
Protein: 0g;
Sodium: 0mg;
Potassium: 150mg;
Phosphorus: 10mg

Direction

1. Warm up your oven to 350deg.F.
2. Wash then core the apples, leaving the bottoms intact.
3. Spray cinnamon evenly over each apple.
4. Spray a small amount of honey over the apples if anticipated.
5. Put your apples in your baking dish and include a little water to the bottom of the dish.
6. Cover the dish using aluminum foil then bake for around 30 mins, or 'til the apples are soft.
7. Present warm.

118 Grilled Pineapple with Honey Drizzle

PREPARATION TIME 5 MIN · COOKING TIME 5 MIN · SERVINGS 2

Ingredients

- 1/2 pineapple, skinned and carved
- 1 tsp honey (elective, use sparingly)

Per serving:
Calories: 70kcal;
Fat: 0g;
Carbs: 18g;
Protein: 1g;
Sodium: 0mg;
Potassium: 140mg;
Phosphorus: 10mg

Direction

1. Warm up grill or your grill pan in a med-high temp.
2. Grill the pineapple slices for 2-3 mins on all sides till they have grill marks.
3. Spray a small amount of honey over the grilled pineapple if anticipated.
4. Present warm as a tasty dessert or snack.

119 Almond and Coconut Macaroons

PREPARATION TIME 15 MIN · COOKING TIME 15 MIN · SERVINGS 4

Ingredients

- 1/2 teacup unsweetened teared up coconut
- 1/4 teacup almond meal (ground almonds)
- 2 egg whites
- 1/4 tsp almond extract (elective)
- Stevia or erythritol (elective, for added sweetness)

Per serving:
Calories: 90kcal;
Fat: 7g;
Carbs: 4g;
Protein: 2g;
Sodium: 10mg;
Potassium: 40mg;
Phosphorus: 20mg

Direction

1. Warm up your oven to 350 deg. F then line your baking sheet using parchment paper.
2. Inside your container, blend the teared up coconut and almond meal.
3. Inside your distinct container, beat the egg whites till they form stiff peaks.
4. Gently wrap the egg whites into your coconut and almond solution.
5. Include almond extract and a small amount of stevia or erythritol if anticipated for sweetness.
6. Drop spoonful of the solution onto your prepared baking sheet.
7. Bake for 12-15 mins or 'til the macaroons are mildly golden.
8. Let them cool prior to serving.

120 Peach Sorbet

Ingredients

PREPARATION TIME 5 MIN
COOKING TIME 0 MIN
SERVINGS 2

- 2 ripe peaches (skinned and eroded)
- 1/2 teacup unsweetened almond milk
- 1/2 tsp vanilla extract
- Stevia or erythritol (elective, for added sweetness)

Per serving:
Calories: 60kcal;
Fat: 1g;
Carbs: 14g;
Protein: 1g;
Sodium: 50mg;
Potassium: 220mg;
Phosphorus: 20mg

Direction

1. Cut the peaches into chunks.
2. Inside a mixer, blend the peach chunks, unsweetened almond milk, and vanilla extract.
3. Blend 'til smooth.
4. Taste then include a small amount of stevia or erythritol if anticipated for sweetness.
5. Pour your solution into a container and freeze for almost 2 hrs.
6. Present as a delightful peach sorbet.

121 Rice Pudding with Raisins

Ingredients

PREPARATION TIME 10 MIN
COOKING TIME 25 MIN
SERVINGS 4

- 1/2 teacup white rice (washed)
- 2 teacups unsweetened almond milk
- 1/4 teacup raisins
- 1/4 tsp ground cinnamon
- Stevia or erythritol (elective, for added sweetness)

Per serving:
Calories: 140kcal;
Fat: 1g;
Carbs: 32g;
Protein: 2g;
Sodium: 100mg;
Potassium: 60mg;
Phosphorus: 40mg

Direction

1. Inside your saucepot, blend the washed rice and almond milk.
2. Boil, lower heat, cover, then simmer for around 20-25 mins, mixing irregularly 'til the rice is soft then the solution thickens.
3. Stir in raisins and ground cinnamon.
4. Cook for an extra 5 mins, or 'til the raisins are plump and the pudding has thickened further.
5. Take outfrom temp., allow it cool mildly, and sweeten with stevia or erythritol if anticipated.
6. Present warm or chilled

122 Lemon Zest Popsicles

Ingredients

PREPARATION TIME **10** MIN | COOKING TIME **0** MIN | SERVINGS **4**

- 1 lemon (zest and juice)
- 2 teacups unsweetened coconut water
- Stevia or erythritol (elective, for added sweetness)

Per serving:
Calories: 10kcal;
Fat: 0g;
Carbs: 3g;
Protein: 0g;
Sodium: 60mg;
Potassium: 140mg;
Phosphorus: 10mg

Direction

1. Inside your container, blend the lemon zest and juice with the unsweetened coconut water.
2. Taste and include stevia or erythritol if you'd like it sweeter.
3. Pour your solution into popsicle molds.
4. Freeze for 4-6 hrs or 'til fully set.
5. Take out from the molds and relish your refreshing lemon zest popsicles.

123 Mixed Berry Compote

Ingredients

PREPARATION TIME **5** MIN | COOKING TIME **10** MIN | SERVINGS **2**

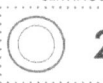

- 1 teacup mixed berries (blueberries, raspberries, strawberries)
- 1/4 teacup water
- 1/4 tsp lemon juice
- Stevia or erythritol (elective, for added sweetness)

Per serving:
Calories: 25kcal;
Fat: 0g;
Carbs: 6g;
Protein: 0g;
Sodium: 0mg;
Potassium: 60mg;
Phosphorus: 10mg

Direction

1. Inside your saucepot, blend the mixed berries, water, and lemon juice.
2. Bring to a simmer in a middling temp.
3. Cook for around 8-10 mins, or 'til the berries break down and the solution thickens.
4. Taste and sweeten with stevia or erythritol if anticipated.
5. Take out from temp. and allow it to cool.
6. Present the mixed berry compote as a topping for yogurt or desserts.

124 Poached Pears with Cinnamon Stick

Ingredients

PREPARATION TIME 10 MIN   COOKING TIME 20 MIN   SERVINGS 2

- 2 ripe pears (skinned and cored)
- 2 teacups water
- 1 cinnamon stick
- Stevia or erythritol (elective, for added sweetness)

Per serving:
Calories: 90kcal;
Fat: 0g;
Carbs: 24g;
Protein: 1g;
Sodium: 10mg;
Potassium: 180mg;
Phosphorus: 20mg

Direction

1. Inside your saucepot, blend the water and cinnamon stick.
2. Include your skinned and cored pears to the saucepan.
3. Bring to a simmer then poach the pears for around 15-20 mins or 'til they are soft when pierced using a fork.
4. Take out your pears from the poaching liquid then let them cool.
5. Sweeten the poaching liquid with stevia or erythritol if anticipated.
6. Present the poached pears sprayd with the sweetened cinnamon-infused liquid.

125 Coconut Rice Pudding

Ingredients

PREPARATION TIME 10 MIN   COOKING TIME 30 MIN   SERVINGS 4

- 1/2 teacup white rice (washed)
- 2 teacups unsweetened coconut milk
- 1/4 teacupteared up coconut
- Stevia or erythritol (elective, for added sweetness)

Per serving:
Calories: 150kcal;
Fat: 9g;
Carbs: 16g;
Protein: 1g;
Sodium: 20mg;
Potassium: 60mg;
Phosphorus: 10mg

Direction

1. Inside your saucepot, blend the washed rice and unsweetened coconut milk.
2. Boil, lower heat, cover, then simmer for around 25-30 mins, mixing irregularly 'til the rice is soft then the solution thickens.
3. Stir in teared up coconut.
4. Cook for an extra 5 mins.
5. Sweeten with stevia or erythritol if anticipated.
6. Present warm or chilled.

126 Berry Gelatin Dessert

Ingredients

PREPARATION TIME 10 MIN   COOKING TIME 0 MIN   SERVINGS 4

- 1 teacup mixed berries (blueberries, raspberries, strawberries)
- 1 teacup unsweetened fruit juice (e.g., apple or cranberry juice)
- 1 packet unflavored gelatin

> **Per serving:**
> Calories: 40kcal;
> Fat: 0g;
> Carbs: 10g;
> Protein: 1g;
> Sodium: 20mg;
> Potassium: 70mg;
> Phosphorus: 5mg

Direction

1. Inside your small saucepan, warm the fruit juice at low heat without boiling.
2. Spray the unflavored gelatin evenly over the juice and allow it to relax for a min to soften.
3. Stir the gelatin till it completely dissolves into your juice.
4. Inside your distinct container, include the mixed berries.
5. Pour your gelatin solution over the berries and stir carefully to blend.
6. Split the solution into serving glasses or molds.
7. Chill in your fridge for 2-3 hrs or 'til set.
8. Present your homemade berry gelatin dessert.

127 Sautéed Apples with Cinnamon

Ingredients

> PREPARATION TIME 10 MIN   COOKING TIME 10 MIN   SERVINGS 2

- 2 apples (choose low-potassium varieties like Granny Smith)
- 1/2 tsp ground cinnamon
- Stevia or erythritol (elective, for added sweetness)

> **Per serving:**
> Calories: 70kcal;
> Fat: 0g;
> Carbs: 19g;
> Protein: 0g;
> Sodium: 0mg;
> Potassium: 110mg;
> Phosphorus: 10mg

Direction

1. Wash, peel, then core the apples, then cut them into slices or chunks.
2. Warm yournon-stick griddle in a middling temp.
3. Include the apple slices and spray with ground cinnamon.
4. Sauté for around 8-10 mins, or 'til the apples are soft and mildly caramelized.
5. Sweeten with stevia or erythritol if anticipated.
6. Present warm as a comforting dessert.

128 Strawberry Rice Crispy Treats

Ingredients

PREPARATION TIME 10 MIN   COOKING TIME 0 MIN   SERVINGS 4

- 2 teacups low-sodium rice cereal
- 1/2 teacup unsweetened applesauce
- 1/2 teacup mashed strawberries
- Stevia or erythritol (elective, for added sweetness)

Per serving:
Calories: 80kcal;
Fat: 0g;
Carbs: 19g;
Protein: 1g;
Sodium: 60mg;
Potassium: 30mg;
Phosphorus: 10mg

Direction

1. Inside a blending container, blend the rice cereal, unsweetened applesauce, and mashed strawberries.
2. Mix till well blended.
3. Sweeten with stevia or erythritol if anticipated.
4. Press the solution into aoiled 8x8-inch pan.
5. Chill in your fridgefor around 30 mins or 'til set.
6. Cut into squares and present your strawberry rice crispy treats.

129 Mango and Coconut Milk Ice Cream

Ingredients

PREPARATION TIME 10 MIN   COOKING TIME 0 MIN   SERVINGS 4

- 2 ripe mangoes, skinned and cubed
- 1 tin (13.5 oz) unsweetened coconut milk
- Stevia or erythritol (elective, for added sweetness)

Per serving:
Calories: 170kcal;
Fat: 16g;
Carbs: 10g;
Protein: 1g;
Sodium: 20mg;
Potassium: 220mg;
Phosphorus: 10mg

Direction

1. Inside a mixer, blend the cubed mangoes and unsweetened coconut milk.
2. Blend 'til smooth.
3. Taste and include stevia or erythritol if anticipated.
4. Pour solution into your ice cream maker then churn using the manufacturer's guidelines.
5. Transfer your churned ice cream to your airtight container and freeze for an extra 2 hrs to firm up.
6. Present yrour homemade mango and coconut milk ice cream.

130 Vanilla Almond Biscotti

Ingredients

PREPARATION TIME 15 MIN COOKING TIME 25 MIN SERVINGS 4

Per serving:
Calories: 110kcal;
Fat: 7g;
Carbs: 6g;
Protein: 5g;
Sodium: 10mg;
Potassium: 30mg;
Phosphorus: 20mg

- 1/2 teacup almond meal (ground almonds)
- 1/4 teacup oat flour (made from oats that are not whole grain)
- 1/4 tsp baking powder
- 1/4 tsp ground cinnamon
- 1/4 tsp vanilla extract
- 1 egg white
- Stevia or erythritol (elective, for added sweetness)

Direction

1. Warm up your oven to 325 deg. F then line your baking sheet using parchment paper.
2. Inside your container, blend almond meal, oat flour, baking powder, and ground cinnamon.
3. Inside your distinct container, whisk collectively the egg white and vanilla extract.
4. Put your wet components to the dry components and mix till a dough forms.
5. Shape the dough into a log shape on the prepared baking sheet.
6. Bake for around 20-25 mins or 'til the biscotti is firm and mildly browned.
7. Let it cool mildly, then slice into biscotti-sized pieces.
8. Optional: sweeten with stevia or erythritol if anticipated.
9. Present your vanilla almond biscotti.

Snacks
and Sides

Recipes

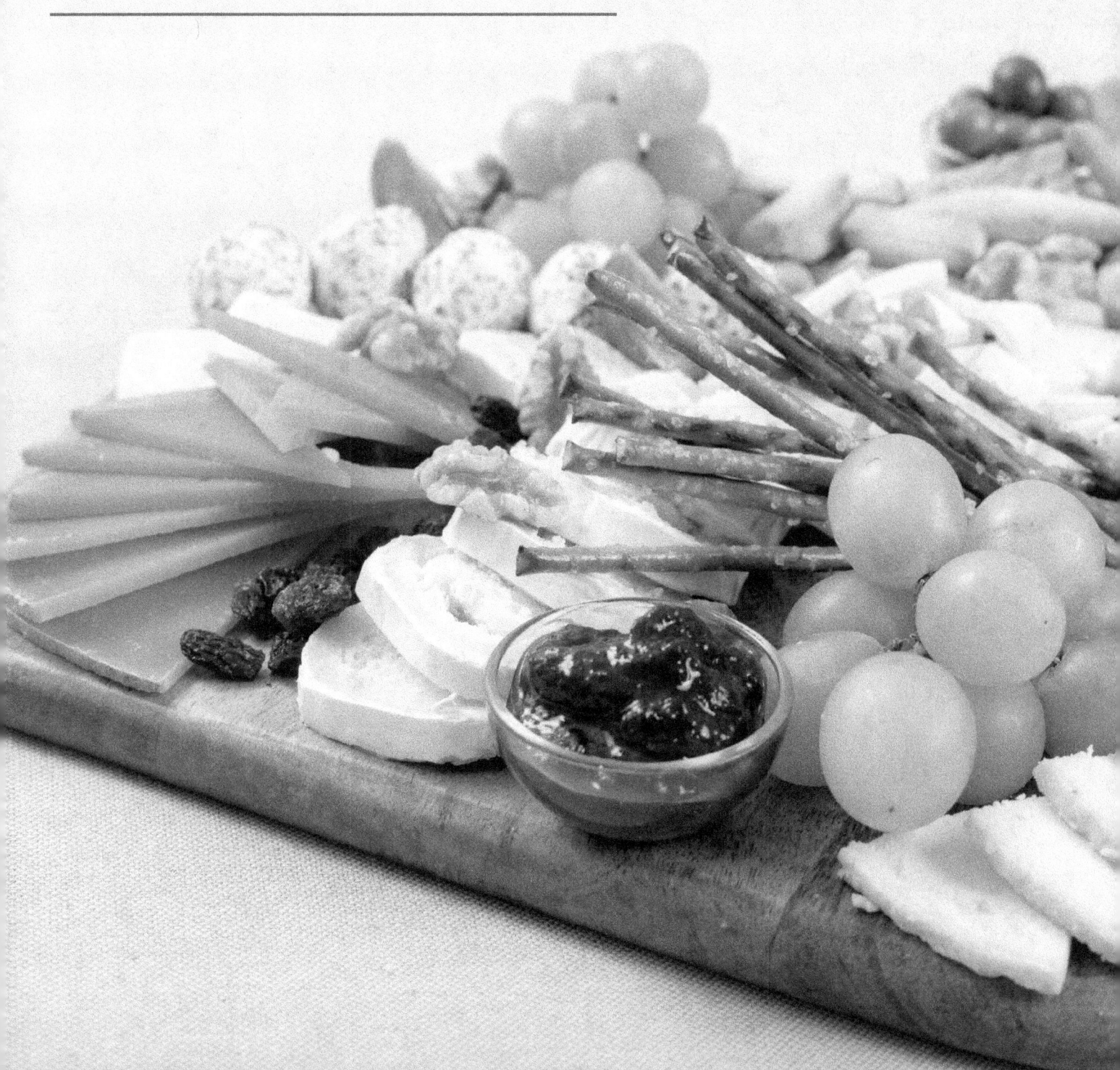

131 Rice Crackers with Cucumber Slices

Ingredients

- 10 rice crackers
- 1/2 cucumber, carved

Per serving:
Calories: 60kcal;
Fat: 0.5g;
Carbs: 13g;
Protein: 1g;
Sodium: 200mg;
Potassium: 100mg;
Phosphorus: 15mg

Direction

1. Simply arrange the rice crackers and cucumber slices on a plate.
2. Relish as a light and crunchy snack.

132 Sautéed Green Beans with Garlic

Ingredients

- 2 teacups fresh green beans, clipped
- 2 pieces garlic, crushed
- 1 tbsp olive oil
- Salt and pepper as needed

Per serving:
Calories: 70kcal;
Fat: 3.5g;
Carbs: 9g;
Protein: 2g;
Sodium: 15mg;
Potassium: 240mg;
Phosphorus: 40mg

Direction

1. Warm olive oil in your pan in a middling temp.
2. Includecrushed garlic and sauté for around 30 secstill fragrant.
3. Include green beans and sauté for around 8-10 mins 'til they are soft-crisp.
4. Flavour using salt and pepper as needed.
5. Present hot.

133 Roasted Red Pepper Hummus with Veggie Sticks

Ingredients

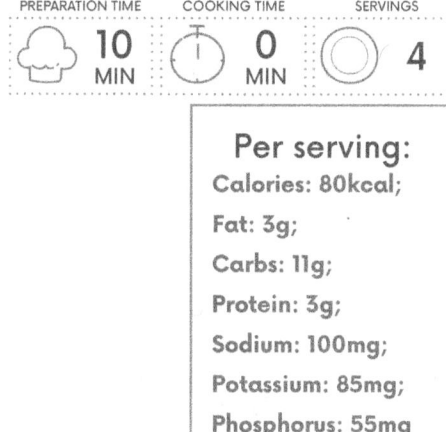

PREPARATION TIME **10** MIN   COOKING TIME **0** MIN   SERVINGS **4**

- 1 tin (15 oz) low-sodium chickpeas, drained and washed
- 1 roasted red pepper
- 1 piece garlic
- 2 tbsps lemon juice
- 1 tbsp olive oil
- Carrot and cucumber sticks for soaking

Per serving:
Calories: 80kcal;
Fat: 3g;
Carbs: 11g;
Protein: 3g;
Sodium: 100mg;
Potassium: 85mg;
Phosphorus: 55mg

Direction

1. Inside your blending container, blend chickpeas, roasted red pepper, garlic, lemon juice, and olive oil.
2. Blend 'til smooth, adding a little water if needed for anticipated uniformity.
3. Present with carrot and cucumber sticks for soaking.

134 Caramelized Onions

Ingredients

PREPARATION TIME **5** MIN   COOKING TIME **20** MIN   SERVINGS **2**

- 1 big onion, finelycarved
- 1 tsp olive oil
- 1 tsp low-sodium vegetable broth (elective)

Per serving:
Calories: 50kcal;
Fat: 1g;
Carbs: 11g;
Protein: 1g;
Sodium: 5mg;
Potassium: 90mg;
Phosphorus: 20mg

Direction

1. Warm olive oil in your griddle in a med-low temp..
2. Include the carved onions then cook, mixing irregularly, for around 20 mins 'til they become soft and caramelized. You can include a tsp of low-sodium vegetable broth if needed to prevent sticking.

135 Rice Cakes with Almond Butter

PREPARATION TIME 5 MIN   COOKING TIME 0 MIN   SERVINGS 2

Ingredients

- 4 rice cakes
- 2 tbsps almond butter (use sparingly)

Per serving:
Calories: 113kcal;
Fat: 5g;
Carbs: 15g;
Protein: 3g;
Sodium: 0mg;
Potassium: 30mg;
Phosphorus: 45mg

Direction

1. Disperse a thin layer of your almond butter on each rice cake.
2. Relish as a simple and satisfying snack.

136 Fresh Pineapple Cubes

PREPARATION TIME 5 MIN   COOKING TIME 0 MIN   SERVINGS 2

Ingredients

- 1 teacup fresh pineapple cubes

Per serving:
Calories: 80kcal;
Fat: 0.2g;
Carbs: 21g;
Protein: 0.9g;
Sodium: 0mg;
Potassium: 180mg;
Phosphorus: 13mg

Direction

1. Simply cube the fresh pineapple and presentinstantly.
2. Relish the sweet and tangy pineapple cubes as a refreshing snack.

137 Sautéed Zucchini and Yellow Squash

Ingredients

PREPARATION TIME 10 MIN | COOKING TIME 10 MIN | SERVINGS 2

- 2 small zucchinis, carved
- 2 small yellow squash, carved
- 1 tbsp olive oil
- Salt and pepper as needed

Per serving:
Calories: 80kcal;
Fat: 7g;
Carbs: 6g;
Protein: 2g;
Sodium: 10mg;
Potassium: 400mg;
Phosphorus: 40mg

Direction

1. Warm olive oil in your griddle in a middling temp.
2. Includecarved zucchini and yellow squash and sauté for around 8-10 mins 'til they are soft.
3. Flavour using salt and pepper as needed.
4. Present hot.

138 Fresh Fruit Salad

Ingredients

PREPARATION TIME 10 MIN | COOKING TIME 0 MIN | SERVINGS 2

- 1 teacup fresh berries (e.g., blueberries, strawberries)
- 1 apple, cubed
- 1 pear, cubed
- 1 kiwi, skinned and carved

Per serving:
Calories: 100kcal;
Fat: 0.5g;
Carbs: 25g;
Protein: 1g;
Sodium: 0mg;
Potassium: 220mg;
Phosphorus: 25mg

Direction

1. Blend the fresh berries, cubed apple, cubed pear, and carved kiwi inside a container.
2. Gently shake the fruits together.
3. Presentinstantly as a delicious and colorful fruit salad.

139 Steamed Asparagus with Lemon

Ingredients

PREPARATION TIME: 5 MIN
COOKING TIME: 10 MIN
SERVINGS: 2

- 1 bunch of asparagus, clipped
- Juice of 1 lemon
- Salt and pepper as needed

Per serving:
Calories: 20kcal;
Fat: 0g;
Carbs: 4g;
Protein: 2g;
Sodium: 0mg;
Potassium: 200mg;
Phosphorus: 40mg

Direction

1. Steam the asparagus for around 7-10 mins 'til they are soft-crisp.
2. Take outfrom temp. then spray with lemon juice.
3. Flavour using salt and pepper as needed.
4. Presentinstantly.

140 Grilled Portobello Mushrooms

Ingredients

PREPARATION TIME: 10 MIN
COOKING TIME: 10 MIN
SERVINGS: 2

- 2 big portobello mushrooms
- 1 tbsp olive oil
- Salt and pepper as needed

Per serving:
Calories: 40kcal;
Fat: 4g;
Carbs: 2g;
Protein: 2g;
Sodium: 10mg;
Potassium: 360mg;
Phosphorus: 40mg

Direction

1. Warm up grill or your grill pan to med-high temp.
2. Brush the portobello mushrooms using olive oil and flavour using salt and pepper.
3. Grill the mushrooms for around 5mins on all sides till they are soft and grill marks appear.
4. Present hot.

141 Roasted Brussels Sprouts with Lemon

Ingredients

PREPARATION TIME 10 MIN | COOKING TIME 25 MIN | SERVINGS 2

- 2 teacups Brussels sprouts, clipped and divided
- 1 tbsp olive oil
- Zest and juice of 1 lemon
- Salt and pepper as needed

Per serving:
Calories: 80kcal;
Fat: 4g;
Carbs: 10g;
Protein: 3g;
Sodium: 28mg;
Potassium: 330mg;
Phosphorus: 70mg

Direction

1. Warm up your oven to 400deg.F.
2. Inside your container, shake the Brussels sprouts using olive oil, lemon zest, salt, and pepper.
3. Disperse your Brussels sprouts on your baking sheet and roast for around 20-25 mins 'til they are soft and mildly crispy.
4. Spray with lemon juice prior to serving.

142 Baked Carrot Sticks with Herbs

Ingredients

PREPARATION TIME 10 MIN | COOKING TIME 20 MIN | SERVINGS 2

- 2 teacups carrot sticks
- 1 tbsp olive oil
- 1 tsp dried herbs (e.g., thyme, rosemary)
- Salt and pepper as needed

Per serving:
Calories: 70kcal;
Fat: 4g;
Carbs: 9g;
Protein: 1g;
Sodium: 60mg;
Potassium: 340mg;
Phosphorus: 30mg

Direction

1. Warm up your oven to 400deg.F.
2. Shake your carrot sticks using olive oil, dried herbs, salt, and pepper.
3. Disperse them on your baking sheet then bake for around 20 mins 'til they are soft and mildly caramelized.
4. Present hot.

143 Boiled Edamame with Sea Salt

Ingredients

- 2 teacups edamame (frozen or fresh)
- Sea salt for seasoning

PREPARATION TIME	COOKING TIME	SERVINGS
5 MIN	5 MIN	2

Per serving:
Calories: 120kcal;
Fat: 5g;
Carbs: 9g;
Protein: 11g;
Sodium: 5mg;
Potassium: 220mg;
Phosphorus: 125mg

Direction

1. Boil the edamame in salted water for around 5mins, or 'til they are soft.
2. Drain your edamame and flavour with a little sea salt.
3. Present as a healthy and protein-rich snack.

144 Cucumber and Radish Slices with Lemon Zest

Ingredients

- 1 cucumber, finelycarved
- 6-8 radishes, finelycarved
- Zest and juice of 1 lemon
- Salt and pepper as needed

PREPARATION TIME	COOKING TIME	SERVINGS
10 MIN	0 MIN	2

Per serving:
Calories: 20kcal;
Fat: 0g;
Carbs: 5g;
Protein: 1g;
Sodium: 20mg;
Potassium: 220mg;
Phosphorus: 15mg

Direction

1. Inside your container, blend the cucumber and radish slices.
2. Put lemon zest, lemon juice, salt, and pepper.
3. Shake to cover evenly.
4. Present as a light and refreshing salad.

145 Cauliflower Rice Pilaf

Ingredients

PREPARATION TIME	COOKING TIME	SERVINGS
10 MIN	25 MIN	2

- 2 teacups cauliflower rice (store-bought or homemade)
- 1 tbsp olive oil
- 1/4 teacupcubed onions
- 1/4 teacupcubed bell peppers
- 1/4 teacupcubed carrots
- 1/4 teacup frozen peas (elective)
- 1/2 tsp dried herbs (e.g., thyme, basil)
- Salt and pepper as needed

Per serving:
Calories: 60kcal;
Fat: 4g;
Carbs: 6g;
Protein: 2g;
Sodium: 30mg;
Potassium: 350mg;
Phosphorus: 40mg

Direction

1. Warm olive oil in your griddle in a middling temp.
2. Includecubed onions, bell peppers, and carrots. Sauté for around 5mins 'til they soften.
3. Include cauliflower rice, frozen peas (if using), dried herbs, salt, and pepper. Cook for an extra 5 mins, mixing irregularly, 'til cauliflower rice is soft.
4. Present as a flavorful rice substitute.

146 Roasted Red Peppers with Herbs

Ingredients

PREPARATION TIME	COOKING TIME	SERVINGS
10 MIN	25 MIN	2

- 2 red bell peppers
- 1 tbsp olive oil
- 1/2 tsp dried herbs (e.g., basil, oregano)
- Salt and pepper as needed

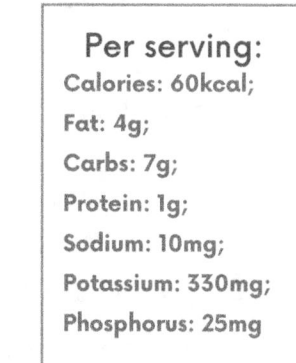

Per serving:
Calories: 60kcal;
Fat: 4g;
Carbs: 7g;
Protein: 1g;
Sodium: 10mg;
Potassium: 330mg;
Phosphorus: 25mg

Direction

1. Warm up your oven to 400deg.F.
2. Cut the red bell peppers into quarters, removing the seeds and membranes.
3. Shake your pepper quarters using olive oil, dried herbs, salt, and pepper.
4. Put on your baking sheet and roast for around 20-25 mins 'til they are soft and mildly caramelized.
5. Present as a delicious side dish.

147 Grilled Eggplant Slices

Ingredients

PREPARATION TIME	10 MIN
COOKING TIME	10 MIN
SERVINGS	2

- 1 big eggplant, carved into rounds
- 1 tbsp olive oil
- Salt and pepper as needed

Per serving:
Calories: 80kcal;
Fat: 4g;
Carbs: 11g;
Protein: 1g;
Sodium: 5mg;
Potassium: 320mg;
Phosphorus: 30mg

Direction

1. Warm up grill or your grill pan to med-high temp.
2. Brush the eggplant slices using olive oil and flavour using salt and pepper.
3. Grill the slices for around 5mins on all sides till they are soft and have grill marks.
4. Present hot.

148 Steamed Broccoli with Garlic

Ingredients

PREPARATION TIME	10 MIN
COOKING TIME	5 MIN
SERVINGS	2

- 2 teacups broccoli florets
- 2 pieces garlic, crushed
- Salt and pepper as needed

Per serving:
Calories: 30kcal;
Fat: 0g;
Carbs: 7g;
Protein: 2g;
Sodium: 20mg;
Potassium: 230mg;
Phosphorus: 45mg

Direction

1. Steam the broccoli florets in your steamer basket for around 5mins 'til they are soft-crisp.
2. Inside your separate small pan, sauté the crushed garlic for around 30 secstill fragrant.
3. Shake your steamed broccoli with the sautéed garlic, and flavour using salt and pepper.
4. Present hot.

149 Sautéed Spinach with Garlic

PREPARATION TIME	COOKING TIME	SERVINGS
5 MIN	5 MIN	2

Ingredients

- · 4 teacups fresh spinach (moderate amount)
- · 2 pieces garlic, crushed
- · 1 tbsp olive oil
- · Salt and pepper as needed

Per serving:
Calories: 50kcal;
Fat: 4g;
Carbs: 3g;
Protein: 2g;
Sodium: 45mg;
Potassium: 400mg;
Phosphorus: 20mg

Direction

1. Warm olive oil in your griddle in a middling temp.
2. Includecrushed garlic and sauté for around 30 secstill fragrant.
3. Include the spinach to the griddle and sauté for 2-3 mins 'til wilted.
4. Flavour using salt and pepper as needed.
5. Present as a nutritious side dish.

150 Baked Butternut Squash with Cinnamon

Ingredients

PREPARATION TIME	COOKING TIME	SERVINGS
10 MIN	30 MIN	2

- 2 teacups butternut squash cubes
- 1 tbsp olive oil
- 1/2 tsp ground cinnamon
- Salt and pepper as needed

Per serving:
Calories: 80kcal;
Fat: 4g;
Carbs: 12g;
Protein: 1g;
Sodium: 5mg;
Potassium: 440mg;
Phosphorus: 30mg

Direction

1. Warm up your oven to 400deg.F.
2. Shake your butternut squash cubes using olive oil, ground cinnamon, salt, and pepper.
3. Disperse them on your baking sheet then bake for around 25-30 mins 'til they are soft and mildly caramelized.
4. Present as a sweet & savory side dish.

Measurement Conversion Table

Volume Equivalents (Liquid)

US Standard	US Standard (oz.)	Metric (approximate)
2 tbsps	1 fl. oz.	30 milliliter
¼ teacup	2 fl. oz.	60 milliliter
½ teacup	4 fl. oz.	120 milliliter
1 teacup	8 fl. oz.	240 milliliter
1½ teacups	12 fl. oz.	355 milliliter
2 teacups or 1 pint	16 fl. oz.	475 milliliter
4 teacups or 1 quart	32 fl. oz.	1 Liter
1 gallon	128 fl. oz.	4 Liter

Volume Equivalents (Dry)

US Standard	Metric (approximate)
⅛ tsp	0.5 milliliter
¼ tsp	1 milliliter
½ tsp	2 milliliter
¾ tsp	4 milliliter
1 tsp	5 milliliter
1 tbsp	15 milliliter
¼ teacup	59 milliliter
⅓ teacup	79 milliliter
½ teacup	118 milliliter
⅔ teacup	156 milliliter
¾ teacup	177 milliliter
1 teacup	235 milliliter
2 teacups or 1 pint	475 milliliter
3 teacups	700 milliliter
4 teacups or 1 quart	1 Liter

Oven Temperatures

Fahrenheit (F)	Celsius (C) (approximate)
250deg.F	120deg.C
300deg.F	150deg.C
325deg.F	165deg.C
350deg.F	180deg.C
375deg.F	190deg.C
400deg.F	200deg.C
425deg.F	220deg.C
450deg.F	230deg.C

Weight Equivalents

US Standard	Metric (approximate)
1 tbsp	15 g
½ oz.	15 g
1 oz.	30 g
2 oz.	60 g
4 oz.	115 g
8 oz.	225 g
12 oz.	340 g
16 oz. or 1 lb.	455 g

30 Days Meal Plan

Day	Breakfast	Lunch	Dinner	Dessert	Nutrition Total
1	10. Veggie Omelet	29. Zucchini and Yellow Squash Soup	58. Balsamic Glazed Roasted Vegetables	118. Grilled Pineapple	Calories: 640kcal Fat: 24g Carbs: 84g Protein: 18g Sodium: 245mg Potassium: 1050mg Phosphorus: 175mg
2	18. Pineapple and Coconut Chia Pudding	36. Zucchini Noodles with Pesto	66. Broiled Sole with Lemon Parsley Sauce	130. Vanilla Almond Biscotti	Calories: 610kcal Fat: 24g Carbs: 96g Protein: 17g Sodium: 160mg Potassium: 1550mg Phosphorus: 265mg
3	3. Vegetable Scrambled Eggs	40. Sautéed Brussels Sprouts with Garlic	75. Grilled Mackerel with Orange Glaze	124. Poached Pears with Cinnamon Stick	Calories: 580kcal Fat: 22g Carbs: 92g Protein: 16g Sodium: 140mg Potassium: 1990mg Phosphorus: 230mg
4	15. Fresh Berry and Rice Milk Smoothie	50. Roasted Cauliflower Steaks	64. Lemon Butter Shrimp	121. Rice Pudding with Raisins	Calories: 600kcal Fat: 22g Carbs: 90g Protein: 16g Sodium: 285mg Potassium: 1290mg Phosphorus: 240mg
5	7. Carrot and Zucchini Muffins	44. Garlic Butter Mushrooms	67. Sautéed Scallops with Garlic	125. Coconut Rice Pudding	Calories: 560kcal Fat: 17g Carbs: 92g Protein: 17g Sodium: 370mg Potassium: 2140mg Phosphorus: 205mg
6	11. Cauliflower Breakfast Hash	52. Stuffed Acorn Squash with Wild Rice	69. Lemon Herb Grilled Trout	129. Mango and Coconut Milk Ice Cream	Calories: 590kcal Fat: 23g Carbs: 100g Protein: 20g Sodium: 170mg Potassium: 2530mg Phosphorus: 230mg
7	6. Cucumber and Egg Breakfast Wrap	58. Balsamic Glazed Roasted Vegetables	62. Pan-seared Cod with Vegetables	127. Sautéed Apples with Cinnamon	Calories: 600kcal Fat: 21g Carbs: 103g Protein: 20g Sodium: 290mg Potassium: 2420mg Phosphorus: 245mg

8	1. Apple Cinnamon Quinoa Porridge	38. Lemon Garlic Sautéed Asparagus	56. Ratatouille with Fresh Basil	122. Lemon Zest Popsicles	Calories: 570kcal Fat: 21g Carbs: 91g Protein: 17g Sodium: 145mg Potassium: 1890mg Phosphorus: 170mg
9	9. Peach Yogurt Parfait	41. Roasted Butternut Squash Cubes	74. Herb-Crusted Tilapia with Lemon	123. Mixed Berry Compote	Calories: 560kcal Fat: 20g Carbs: 95g Protein: 18g Sodium: 155mg Potassium: 1870mg Phosphorus: 220mg
10	16. Pear and Cinnamon Breakfast Rice	48. Cabbage and Carrot Slaw	81. Lemon Herb Grilled Chicken	128. Strawberry Rice Crispy Treats	Calories: 580kcal Fat: 22g Carbs: 95g Protein: 18g Sodium: 165mg Potassium: 2080mg Phosphorus: 225mg
11	5. Pineapple Mint Smoothie	49. Sautéed Green Beans with Almonds	77. Seared Tuna with Avocado Salad	120. Peach Sorbet	Calories: 570kcal Fat: 19g Carbs: 87g Protein: 19g Sodium: 295mg Potassium: 1970mg Phosphorus: 245mg
12	17. Spinach and Egg White Scramble	45. Roasted Beets with Orange Glaze	82. Baked Turkey Breast with Herbs	126. Berry Gelatin Dessert	Calories: 560kcal Fat: 17g Carbs: 95g Protein: 18g Sodium: 275mg Potassium: 2290mg Phosphorus: 220mg
13	20. Rice and Almond Breakfast Pudding	47. Lemon Herb Grilled Zucchini	80. Pan-seared Halibut with Mango Salsa	119. Almond and Coconut Macaroons	Calories: 580kcal Fat: 23g Carbs: 91g Protein: 20g Sodium: 195mg Potassium: 2920mg Phosphorus: 220mg
14	16. Pear and Cinnamon Breakfast Rice	36. Zucchini Noodles with Pesto	86. Chicken Kabobs with Vegetables	128. Strawberry Rice Crispy Treats	Calories: 590kcal Fat: 13g Carbs: 99g Protein: 23g Sodium: 280mg Potassium: 1190mg Phosphorus: 190mg
15	14. Lemon and Blueberry Rice Cakes	37. Cauliflower Fried Rice	60. Avocado and Cucumber Sushi Rolls	124. Poached Pears with Cinnamon Stick	Calories: 510kcal Fat: 11g Carbs: 99g Protein: 14g Sodium: 295mg Potassium: 1420mg Phosphorus: 210mg

16	11. Cauliflower Breakfast Hash	38. Lemon Garlic Sautéed Asparagus	82. Baked Turkey Breast with Herbs	129. Mango and Coconut Milk Ice Cream	Calories: 570kcal Fat: 18g Carbs: 131g Protein: 24g Sodium: 350mg Potassium: 1650mg Phosphorus: 220mg
17	7. Carrot and Zucchini Muffins	39. Roasted Red Peppers Stuffed with Quinoa	68. Baked Haddock with Roasted Vegetables	130. Vanilla Almond Biscotti	Calories: 590kcal Fat: 20g Carbs: 127g Protein: 16g Sodium: 255mg Potassium: 1760mg Phosphorus: 260mg
18	18. Pineapple and Coconut Chia Pudding	40. Sautéed Brussels Sprouts with Garlic	87. Balsamic Glazed Chicken Breast	126. Berry Gelatin Dessert	Calories: 530kcal Fat: 20g Carbs: 124g Protein: 20g Sodium: 355mg Potassium: 1450mg Phosphorus: 185mg
19	3. Vegetable Scrambled Eggs	41. Roasted Butternut Squash Cubes	53. Grilled Mackerel with Orange Glaze	125. Coconut Rice Pudding	Calories: 580kcal Fat: 18g Carbs: 126g Protein: 19g Sodium: 390mg Potassium: 1440mg Phosphorus: 225mg
20	19. Warm Millet Bowl with Fresh Berries	42. Cilantro Lime Cauliflower Rice	83. Pork Tenderloin with Apples	117. Baked Apples with Cinnamon	Calories: 610kcal Fat: 18g Carbs: 137g Protein: 16g Sodium: 345mg Potassium: 1600mg Phosphorus: 245mg
21	5. Pineapple Mint Smoothie	43. Eggplant and Bell Pepper Stir Fry	55. Stuffed Bell Peppers with Rice and Veggies	123. Mixed Berry Compote	Calories: 590kcal Fat: 19g Carbs: 136g Protein: 15g Sodium: 395mg Potassium: 1570mg Phosphorus: 240mg
22	2. Blueberry Rice Pancakes	44. Garlic Butter Mushrooms	58. Balsamic Glazed Roasted Vegetables	121. Rice Pudding with Raisins	Calories: 590kcal Fat: 19g Carbs: 136g Protein: 14g Sodium: 405mg Potassium: 1470mg Phosphorus: 240mg
23	8. Rice Cereal with Sliced Pears	45. Roasted Beets with Orange Glaze	50. Roasted Cauliflower Steaks	118. Grilled Pineapple with Honey Drizzle	Calories: 560kcal Fat: 16g Carbs: 122g Protein: 14g Sodium: 225mg Potassium: 1740mg Phosphorus: 210mg

24	17. Spinach and Egg White Scramble	46. Steamed Artichokes with Olive Oil	76. Baked Catfish with Cajun Spice	122. Lemon Zest Popsicles	Calories: 520kcal Fat: 12g Carbs: 121g Protein: 12g Sodium: 380mg Potassium: 1310mg Phosphorus: 170mg
25	9. Peach Yogurt Parfait	47. Lemon Herb Grilled Zucchini	84. Grilled Lamb Chops with Rosemary	119. Almond and Coconut Macaroons	Calories: 540kcal Fat: 17g Carbs: 113g Protein: 16g Sodium: 180mg Potassium: 1610mg Phosphorus: 180mg
26	4. Rice Flour Waffles with Fresh Berries	48. Cabbage and Carrot Slaw	95. Skillet Chicken with Lemon and Olives	120. Peach Sorbet	Calories: 580kcal Fat: 20g Carbs: 115g Protein: 16g Sodium: 275mg Potassium: 1570mg Phosphorus: 190mg
27	6. Cucumber and Egg Breakfast Wrap	30. White Fish and Veggie Soup	41. Roasted Butternut Squash Cubes	121. Rice Pudding with Raisins	Calories: 610kcal Fat: 15g Carbs: 92g Protein: 17g Sodium: 200mg Potassium: 880mg Phosphorus: 290mg
28	15. Fresh Berry and Rice Milk Smoothie	27. Pumpkin and Sage Soup	68. Baked Haddock with Roasted Vegetables	128. Strawberry Rice Crispy Treats	Calories: 570kcal Fat: 13g Carbs: 89g Protein: 15g Sodium: 185mg Potassium: 890mg Phosphorus: 290mg
29	32. Lemon and Coriander Soup	42. Cilantro Lime Cauliflower Rice	75. Grilled Mackerel with Orange Glaze	124. Poached Pears with Cinnamon Stick	Calories: 560kcal Fat: 12g Carbs: 97g Protein: 24g Sodium: 190mg Potassium: 980mg Phosphorus: 295mg
30	4. Rice Flour Waffles with Fresh Berries	37. Cauliflower Fried Rice	59. Quinoa Stuffed Eggplants	123. Mixed Berry Compote	Calories: 660kcal Fat: 12g Carbs: 141g Protein: 20g Sodium: 195mg Potassium: 1380mg Phosphorus: 275mg